MODERN

REFLEXOLOGY

CASS & JANIE JACKSON

Acknowledgments

Photography: Charles Walker Picture Library p. 16, 28 and 54

Published in 2002 by Caxton Editions

20 Bloomsbury Street

London WC1B 3JH

a member of the Caxton Publishing Group

© 2002 Caxton Publishing Group

Designed and produced for Caxton Editions

by Open Door Limited

Rutland, United Kingdom

Editing: Mary Morton

Typesetting: Jane Booth

Title: Modern Reflexology

ISBN: 1 84067 287 0

MODERN

REFLEXOLOGY

CASS & JANIE JACKSON

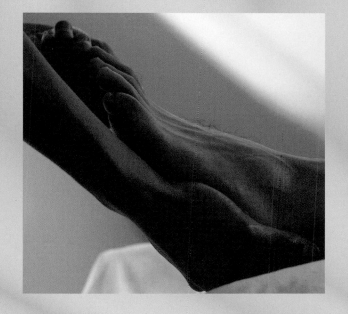

CAXTON EDITIONS

CONTENTS

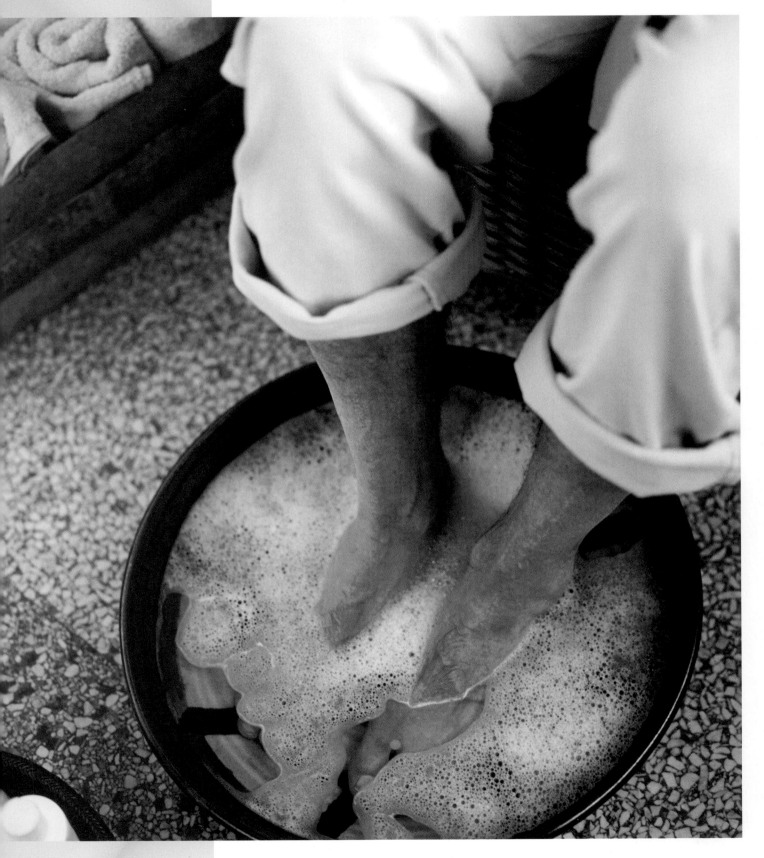

CONTENTS

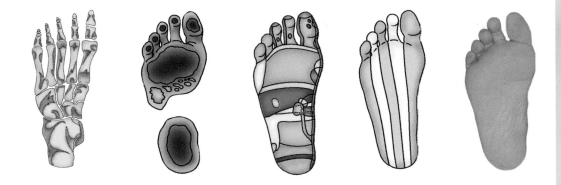

REFLEXOLOGY

INTRODUCTION

At the beginning of the 21st century, health is headline news. There was a time when only hypochondriacs were much concerned with their health. A few years ago, though, attitudes started to change. At first it was merely a fashionable fad to take up jogging or to work out at a gym. Then we noticed that exercise not only made us feel better – we looked better, too. And suddenly, we didn't need pills from the chemist to make us feel good.

From such small beginnings grew the current soaring interest in health. Our concern is not solely with physical well-being. More and more of us recognise that in order to achieve a truly healthy lifestyle we need to consider the whole person – body, mind and spirit. This holistic approach is offered by most of the complementary therapies which are now so widely used. Yoga, aromatherapy, flower remedies, crystal healing and many others offer an escape from Public Enemy No 1 – STRESS.

Below: exercise not only made us feel better – we looked better, too

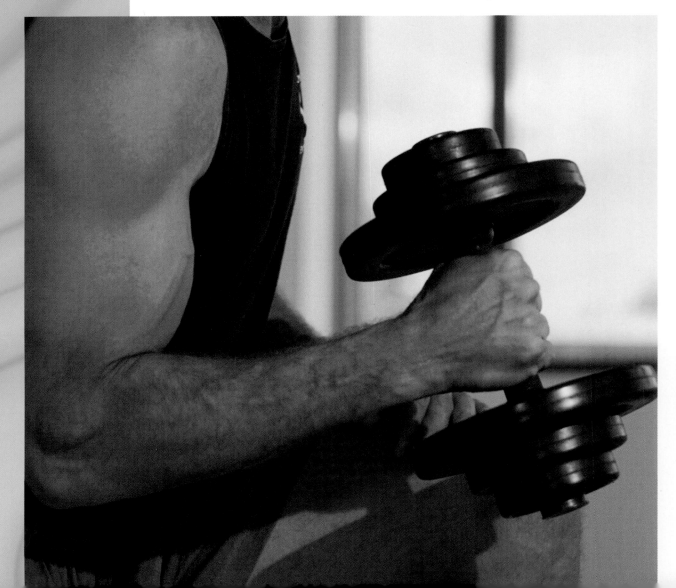

WHAT IS REFLEXOLOGY?

If you're constantly exhausted, have backache and feel unhappy in your work, you're probably suffering from that Millennium malady – stress. It's generally agreed that around 70 per cent of all hospital beds are occupied by patients suffering from stress-related illness. If you'd rather not join their numbers, perhaps a series of reflexology treatments would help.

Thousands of years ago, the Chinese discovered that energy circulates throughout our bodies in channels described as "meridians". In order to stimulate this energy and remove blockages, they applied fine needles at certain points along the meridian pathways. This system is called acupuncture. Acupressure, as its name implies, uses pressure rather than needles. Reflexology, too, is a similar form of treatment, but it concentrates on the feet.

They claim that among the thousands of nerve endings on the sole of each foot, there are "reflex areas", corresponding to every part of your body.

Below: the Chinese claim that there are reflex arecs on the sole of each foot corresponding to everypart of your body.

Below: how can manipulation of the big toe, for example, ease pain in the neck?

During treatment the practitioner can pinpoint "tender reflexes" which indicate that the equivalent body part is under some stress or that energy is blocked. Massage and gentle pressure applied to these points stimulates healing.

Some people feel a bit cynical about this concept. How can manipulation of the big toe, for example, ease pain in the neck? To be fair, it does seem a little far-fetched to claim that foot massage can boost your energy, ease pain in your back, and offer a new angle on problems at the office. Yet reflexology treatment is often found to do all these things and help a number of other health problems.

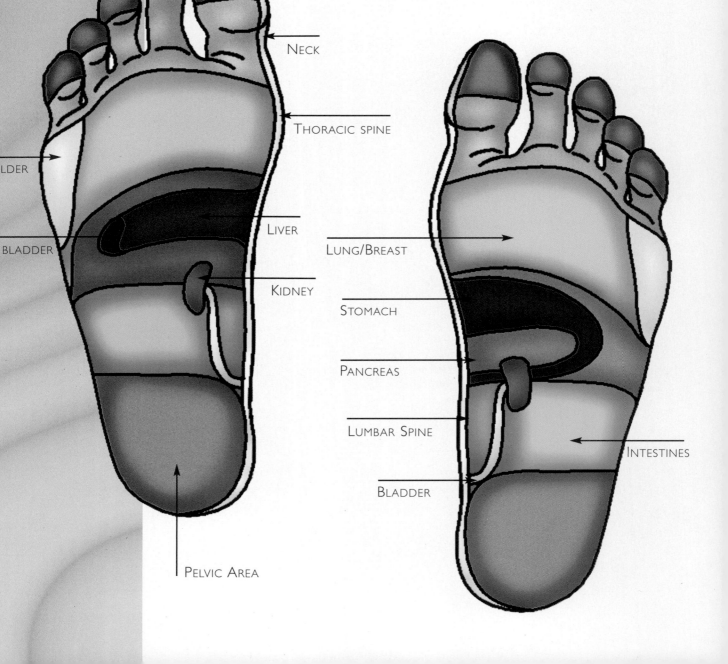

BRAIN

NECK

THORACIC SPINE

SHOULDER

LIVER

LUNG/BREAST

GALL BLADDER

KIDNEY

STOMACH

PANCREAS

LUMBAR SPINE

INTESTINES

BLADDER

PELVIC AREA

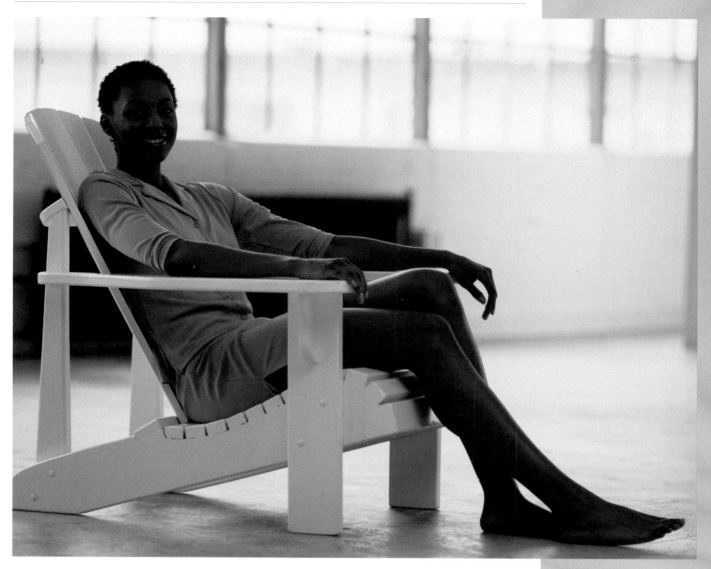

Reflexology is an essentially holistic approach to healing. It aims to treat the whole person – body, mind and spirit – in direct contrast to the specialisation favoured by orthodox medicine. A practitioner will never offer a diagnosis of any problem or promise a cure. Instead, he will aim to "balance" the whole person, thereby creating relaxation and promoting a feeling of well-being.

Such balance is essential to good health, but it can be achieved only when the energy flow throughout the body is unimpeded. Reflexologists believe that stimulation of the pressure points on the feet can clear blockages and facilitate the flow of what the Chinese call the life force.

Above: a practitioner will aim to "balance" the whole person, thereby creating relaxation and promoting a feeling of well-being.

HOW IT ALL BEGAN

As long ago as the 4th century BC reflexology, acupuncture and acupressure were being practised in China. Since Chinese doctors were paid only if the patient recovered, it would seem that all three treatments were found to be effective.

Even further back in history, a form of reflexology was used in Ancient Egypt.

Evidence for this comes from a painting discovered in a tomb at Saqqara, south of Cairo. Dated around 2500–2330 BC the painting depicts two patients receiving some form of foot treatment from the eminent physician Ankmahor and his assistant.

The hieroglyphs explaining the picture indicate that the patient is asking the therapist not to hurt him. This patient, too, has placed his hand under his arm, to show where he feels pain. The physician is apparently applying pressure to the corresponding reflex area on his foot.

Claims that reflexology was practised by the Incas, who passed it on to North American Indians, are unproven. But to this day, members of the Cherokee tribe believe that our feet

Right: a form of reflexology was used in Ancient Egypt.

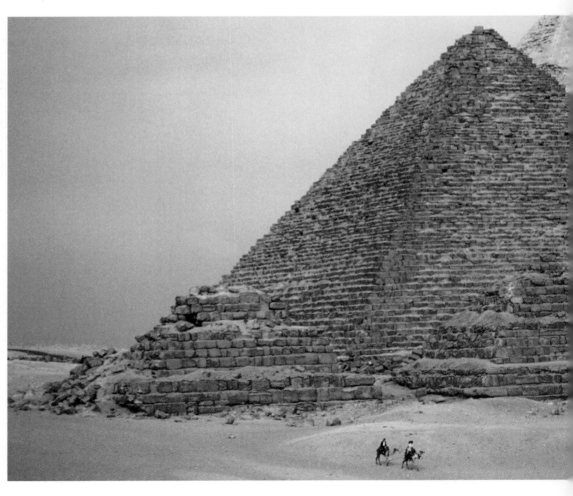

are our contact with the earth and its energies. Perhaps this is the origin of the popular phrase "keeping both feet on the ground".

Some form of pressure therapy is thought to have been practised by African tribes. It was also found in Europe in the 14th and 15th centuries. At that time two eminent physicians, Dr Adamus and Dr A'tatis, suggested that the body could be divided into zones, and treated accordingly. Their book on the subject was published in 1582. However, it seems that little attention was paid to these ideas and they were largely ignored.

During the 19th century, there was more investigation into reflex therapy. In London, Sir Henry Head discovered that some areas of the skin reacted to pressure when organs corresponding to those areas of skin were diseased. The Russians, too, were investigating similar phenomena. For instance, the famous Ivan Pavlov used dogs to advance his theories of conditioned reflexes.

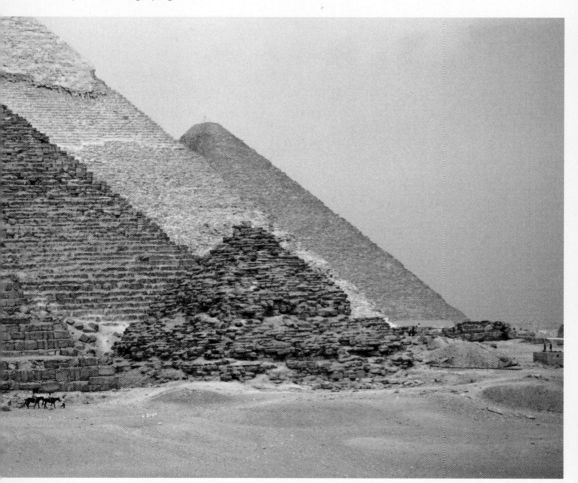

Right: drastic measures, perhaps, but the sceptics were quickly convinced when they felt no pain from the pin prick.

Then, in the 1890s, German doctors developed what they called "reflex massage" as a means of treating disease.

The next "big name" in reflexology is Dr Alfons Cornelius. In 1893 the good doctor was ill. During his convalescence he attended a spa and received massage treatment. One of the therapists seemed to get particularly good results, and Cornelius noted that this man concentrated his efforts mainly on painful areas. Within four weeks, Cornelius was cured. Subsequently, he experimented with the use of pressure on his own patients and in 1902 he published *Pressure Points: The Origin and Significance*.

It is uncertain whether Dr William Fitzgerald ever read this book. Certainly this American ear, nose and throat specialist had visited Europe on a number of occasions and could well have encountered Dr Cornelius. But it was while he was working in America that Fitzgerald discovered, quite by chance, that when pressure was applied to one area of the body, pain was alleviated elsewhere. Intrigued, he investigated further, and proved that discomfort in one area of a certain zone could be eased by pressure on another point in the same zone. The result was the procedure he called "zone therapy".

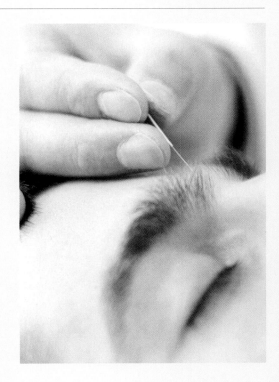

Basically, he divided the body into ten vertical zones, as had the two European doctors, 400 years earlier. This system is still widely used. Each zone is of equal width, and extends from the tips of the toes to the top of the head.

Fitzgerald and his friend Dr. Edwin Bowers were excited about this discovery. Some of their colleagues were less enthusiastic, though, so the two men devised a method of proving the possibilities of zone therapy. Taking the doubting Thomas's hand, they applied pressure to it. Then they stuck a pin in that part of the face which corresponded to the pressure point. Drastic measures, perhaps, but the sceptics were quickly convinced when they felt no pain from the pin prick.

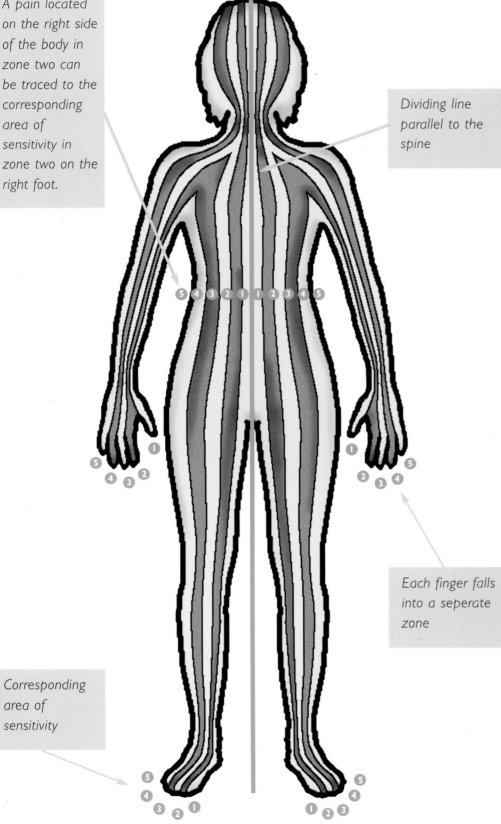

A pain located on the right side of the body in zone two can be traced to the corresponding area of sensitivity in zone two on the right foot.

Dividing line parallel to the spine

Each finger falls into a seperate zone

Corresponding area of sensitivity

Left: zone therapy - Each zone is of equal width, and extends from the tips of the toes to the top of the head.

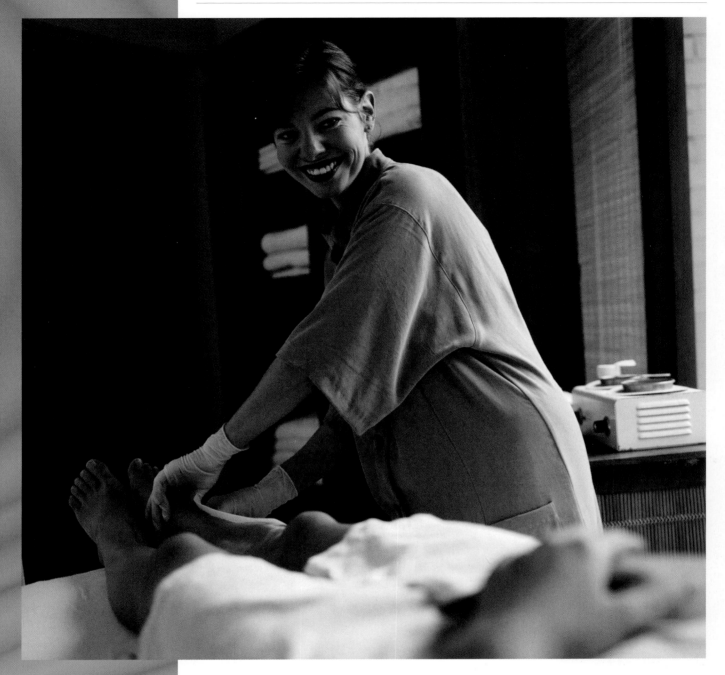

Above: chiropodists, physiotherapists, osteopaths – and many ordinary people – learned Eunice Ingham's technique; reflexology as we know it today had arrived.

Dr Joseph Shelby Riley did not demand proof. It was he, indeed, who introduced the theory to his assistant Eunice Ingham, a physiotherapist. A keen advocate of Fitzgerald's methods, she took his discovery a step further.

Recognising the acute sensitivity of the feet, she charted on them the ten zones of the body. It was she who realised that the shape of the foot was akin to that of the body and offered, in effect, a map of all the body parts and organs.

Ingham used her revolutionary system to treat her own patients, to such good effect that she felt the time had come to go public with the therapy she had christened reflexology. Not only medical practitioners were impressed. People like chiropodists, physiotherapists, osteopaths – and many ordinary people – learned her technique. Reflexology as we know it today had arrived.

It was introduced to the UK in 1960 by one of Ingham's students, Doreen Bayley. Since then, as interest in complementary therapies has increased, it has also become accepted in Australia, New Zealand and most countries throughout the world.

So how does reflexology work?

Below: the complex bones of the human foot.

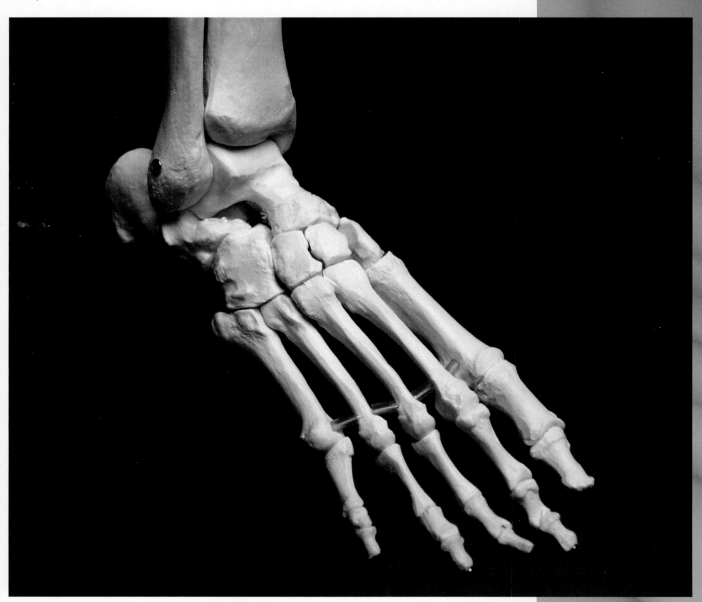

HOW DOES REFLEXOLOGY WORK?

Paracelsus, the 16th-century physician, suggested "A doctor must seek out old wives, gypsies, sorcerers, wandering tribes, old robbers and other such outlaws, and take lessons from them." Today, few orthodox western doctors would agree with his advice. Any treatment not conforming to accepted medical practice is at worst condemned and at best regarded with suspicion. Despite the growing conviction, even in medical circles, that we cannot separate body, mind and spirit, the holistic approach is still not fully accepted. Yet it forms the foundation for many increasingly popular complementary treatments, including reflexology.

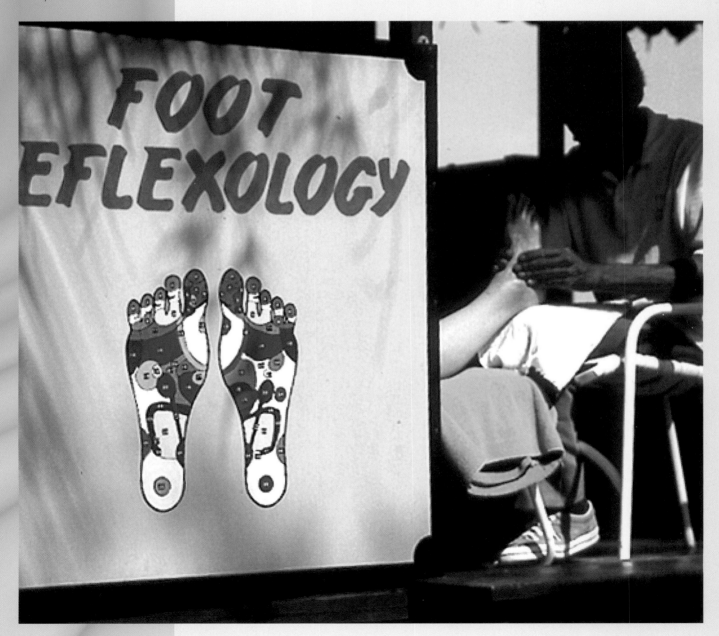

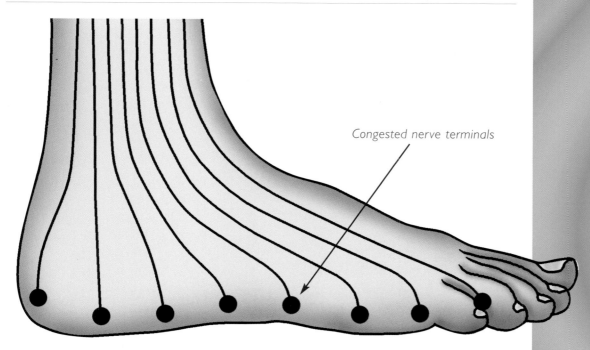

Congested nerve terminals

Little scientific research has been done on exactly how reflexology works. There are a number of theories about it, none of which has yet been proven. But, despite this lack of clinical evidence, there is no suggestion that reflexology is harmful in any way. However, even the most sceptical of critics agree that some aspects of the treatment must be beneficial.

The thousands of nerve endings in the soles of your feet communicate with all areas of your body and brain. That fact is scientifically acknowledged. During reflexology treatment, gentle pressure stimulates those nerve endings and influences all body systems. Massage increases circulation in the feet. This, in turn, enables the blood to distribute nutrients throughout the body and dispose of toxins. Immediately after treatment, you may feel either deeply relaxed or completely rejuvenated. You will certainly feel better, though sometimes – but not always – your condition could appear to worsen next day. If this happens, there's no need to worry. This reaction will be brief.

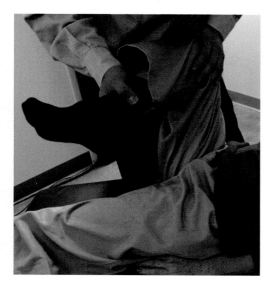

Above: during reflexology treatment, gentle pressure stimulates those nerve endings and influences all body systems.

Right: reflexologists work via ten vertical zones and three transverse zones.

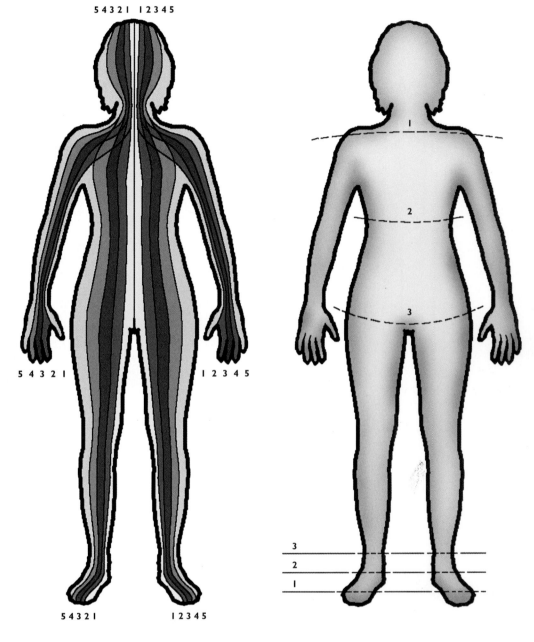

ZONE THERAPY

Reflexology treatment can kick-start your own healing powers and stimulate the energy flow throughout your body.

To do this, reflexologists work via ten vertical zones which, according to Dr Fitzgerald, extend throughout the body from the top of the head to the tips of the fingers and toes, and from front to back. There are five such zones on the left of the body and five on the right, each of equal width.

Additionally, three transverse zones divide the body into four sections.

It is essential to our good health that the energy flow through these zones is maintained. Congestion can occur when waste products such as calcium crystals or uric acid accumulate. When this happens, the practitioner can feel "gritty" patches beneath the skin of your foot. He needs to break down this waste matter to allow the circulation and the lymphatic systems to clear your energy pathways.

KIRLIAN PHOTOGRAPHY

Proof that such clearance does happen is given by the use of Kirlian photography. It is known that human beings, like animals and plants, are surrounded by fields of electrical energy which reflect their physical and emotional health. These "auras" or "halos" can sometimes be observed by those of us who are particularly sensitive or psychic. Kirlian photography reveals these energy fields on film as colours or patterns surrounding the body. Any imbalance is indicated by a halo that is restricted, irregular and muddy. After reflexology treatment, the colours are brighter and the pattern more regular.

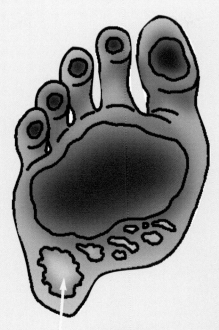
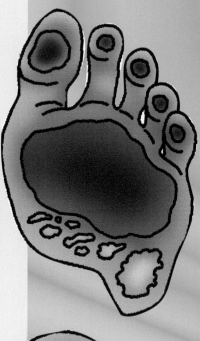
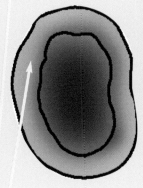
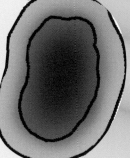

Left: Kirlian photography reveals these energy fields on film as colours or patterns surrounding the body.

Kirlian researchers claim to be able to diagnose both the physical and emotional state of the body by the colours produced in the photograph and their intensity

ENERGY

So what is this energy that plays such an important part in determining our health? It goes by many names. In Japan it's known as ki. The Chinese call it ch'i. In India it is referred to as prana and Tibetans refer to it as lung-gom. We in the west prefer more scientific terminology such as bioplasma.

Below: energy - no matter what it is called, this energy is, quite simply, the Life Force. Without it, we die.

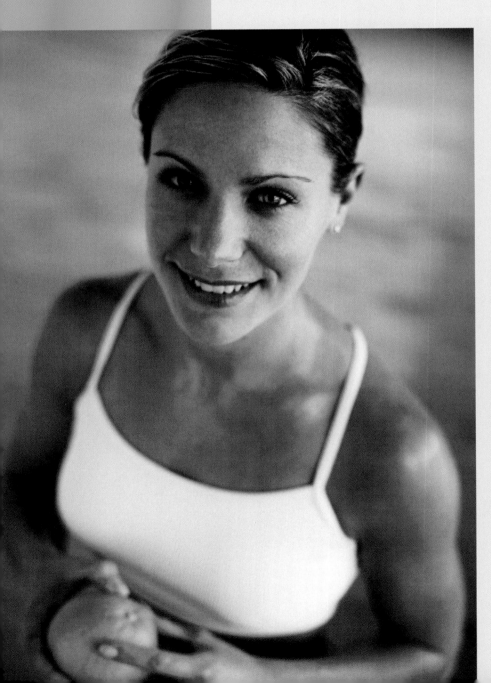

No matter what it is called, this energy is, quite simply, the Life Force. Without it, we die.

All the organs and body parts are linked by a network of channels. The Chinese call these pathways meridians, but to the reflexologist they are known as zones.

In a healthy body, the energy flows freely through these channels, but if blockages exist dis-ease can result.

The word *disease* is deliberately hyphenated. It is not used in the usual way – to denote disease as an ailment. In this context, it is used to indicate that the body or some particular part of it is not at ease with itself. If this type of imbalance or lack of energy continues for any length of time illness is the almost inevitable result, thus – we refer to dis-ease.

STRUCTURE OF THE FOOT

Leonardo da Vinci described the human foot as "A masterpiece of engineering and a work of art." Certainly it is extremely complex, comprising 26 small bones, 20 muscles, 114 ligaments, nerves, blood vessels, connective tissues and – of course – skin.

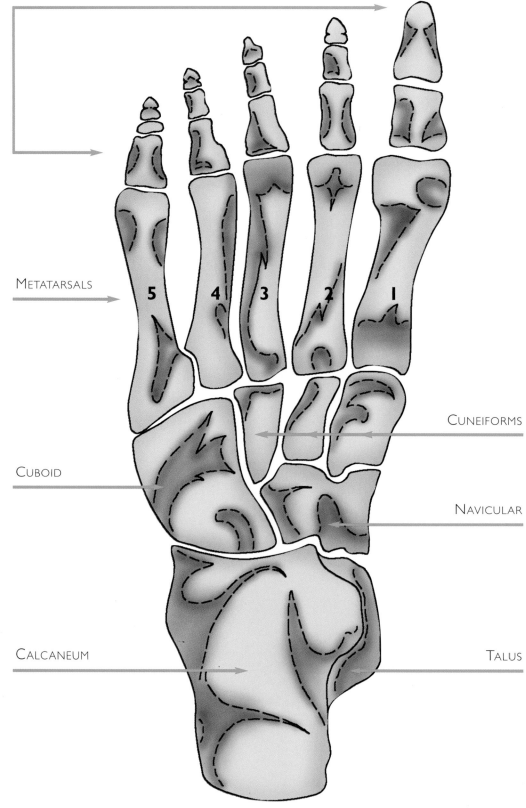

PHALANGES

METATARSALS

5   4   3   2   1

CUBOID

CALCANEUM

CUNEIFORMS

NAVICULAR

TALUS

Left: structure of the Foot - "a masterpiece of engineering and a work of art."

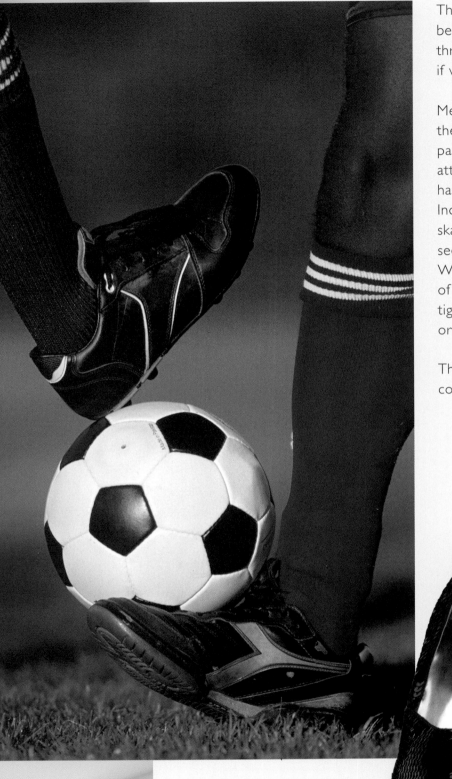

This fragile and intricate structure bears our weight throughout our three score years and ten – or longer, if we are lucky.

Mercifully, the Chinese habit of binding the feet of girl babies belongs to the past. Even so, few of us give as much attention to our feet as we do to our hands and other parts of the anatomy. Indeed, people like ballet dancers, ice skaters, and professional footballers seem intent on ruining their feet. Women are the worst culprits. Slaves of fashion, they cram their feet into tight shoes with ridiculously high heels or platform soles.

Then, after years of such neglect, they complain "My feet are killing me!"

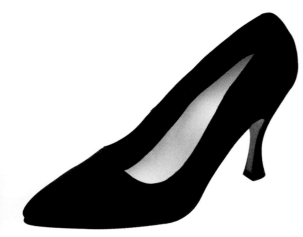

Only when their feet hurt do they really look at them. Then they bewail the ugliness of the hard skin, corns, bunions and ingrowing toenails they see.

Even glamorous film stars, happy to exhibit practically every inch of their bodies, often need to employ a "stand in" for foot photographs.

Foot deformities are not only unsightly and painful, though. Reflexologists believe that they can often be a symptom of dis-ease in other parts of the body. For example, though ill-fitting shoes are the most common cause for bunions, there is evidence to suggest that they may also indicate thyroid trouble. In order to understand this admittedly surprising claim, we need to examine the basic theory of reflexology.

Far left: people like ballet dancers, ice skaters, and professional footballers seem intent on ruining their feet.

Left: film stars, happy to exhibit practically every inch of their bodies, often need to employ a "stand in" for foot photographs.

Right: the ten-zone theory applied to the feet.

Below: reflex points on the soles of the feet

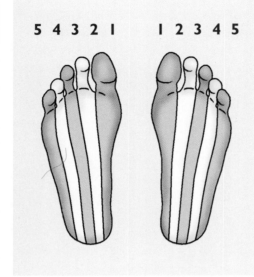

REFLEXES

It was Eunice Ingham who first discovered that Dr Fitzgerald's ten zone theory could be applied to the feet.

Recognising that the shape of the foot closely follows that of the torso, she also realised that each organ and body part is reflected in the feet as a tiny reflex point, located in a similar area on the feet to the position it has in the body.

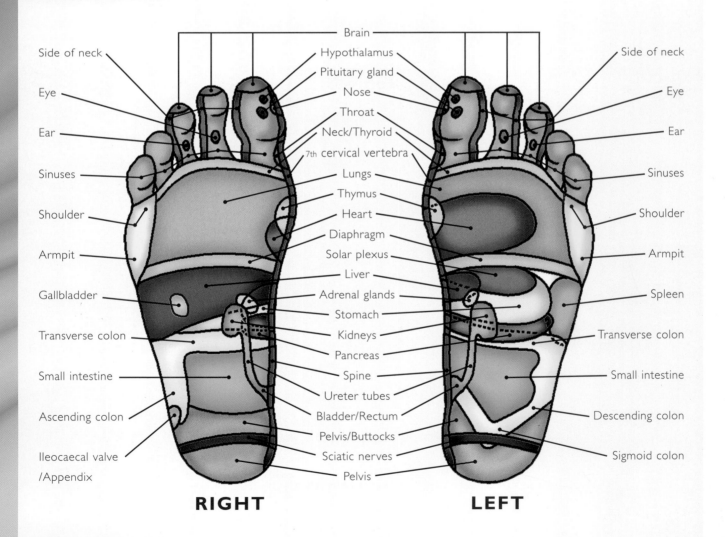

RIGHT   LEFT

Thus, regarding our previous statement that a bunion could be a symptom of problems elsewhere in the body, you will see on the chart that the distortion appears at the same place on the foot as the thyroid reflex point.

In a reflexology treatment, the practitioner's main concern is to establish a state of balance in body, mind and spirit for his client. This happy state is impossible if any aspect of the whole person is not working efficiently. Mental or emotional stress creates an imbalance which can cause physical pain, with resulting dis-ease in the relevant area of the body. Conversely, the tension or discomfort of a physical problem increases mental and emotional stress. Careful examination of the feet can indicate where healing may be required.

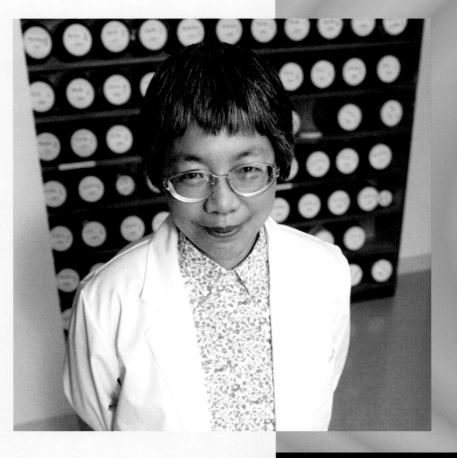

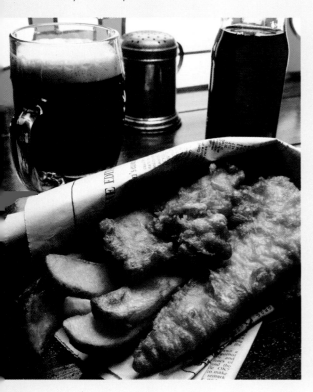

All too often we are ourselves responsible if our bodies are out of balance. If we allow negative attitudes like jealousy, anger, worry, and fear into our lives, they will eventually damage our physical well-being. Lack of exercise and fresh air, a poor diet, heavy smoking and drug or alcohol abuse will have similar effects. A reflexologist can help you to overcome the damage you have inflicted on yourself, but you have an important contribution to make, too. Your restoration to full health is dependent on "combined ops" – a close co-operation between the reflexologist and the person being treated.

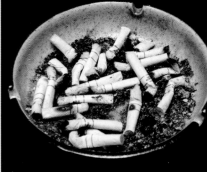

Above: the practitioner's main concern is to establish a state of balance in body, mind and spirit for his client

Left: a poor diet, heavy smoking and drug or alcohol abuse will damage our well-being.

REFLEXOLOGY TECHNIQUES

Right: the tips of fingers or thumbs are used for the rotation technique.

There's much more to reflexology than simply having your feet massaged. In this context, the word "massage" is used loosely and refers to several specialist techniques. During treatment, you will notice that the reflexologist uses his thumb and fingers most of the time. In fact, one of his hands will have a mainly supporting role in holding your foot still to ensure your comfort while he works on the reflex points.

When your therapist is locating these points, he will probe the reflex areas on your feet, in search of particularly sensitive spots. For this exploration, he may use fingers or thumbs.

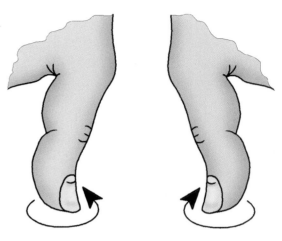

In actually treating the sensitive reflex points, only one thumb will be used, bent at an angle of 45 degrees with the pad against the skin. Your practitioner will apply pressure with the side and end of his thumb, maintaining the bent position. When moving from one point to another, it is rocked gently on to its tip, then stretched out to the next point. It is always in contact with the skin, but you will notice that no pressure is used when the thumb is moving. This technique is known as **caterpillar walking**.

Below: caterpillar walking using the thumb.

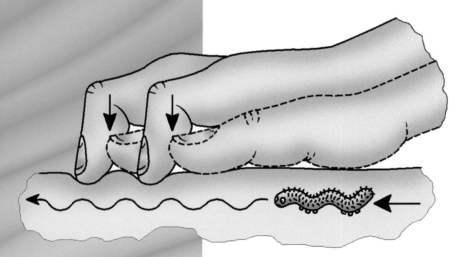

Finger walking is a similar technique, but it is carried out by the side of the index finger. You'll probably find that your therapist will use this on bony areas like the ankle.

The tips of fingers or thumbs are used for the **rotation technique**. When these are gently rotated on the reflex areas, you will feel a slight vibration.

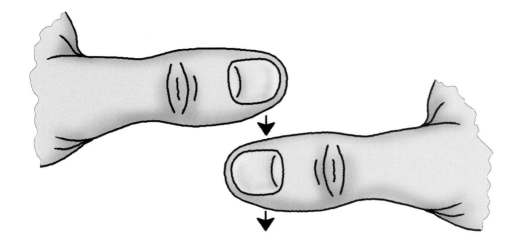

After using either of these techniques, your practitioner is likely to employ the **milking movement**, which helps to flush toxins through the lymphatic system. Placing thumbs or fingers lightly on the reflexes, he will apply slight forward pressure, either in a long continuous movement or in shorter progressive strokes.

The **feathering movement** uses both thumbs or two fingers. Your reflexologist will brush the skin surface, very gently, with one finger or thumb, followed by the other. He will use only the lightest of touches, producing an effect almost like the gentle flow of cool water. Some practitioners use this technique to conclude each part of the treatment.

Don't be alarmed if you see your practitioner clench his fist. He's about to **knead** your foot. In this technique, he will apply the flat side of the clenched fist on the arch area of the sole of your foot. At the same time, he will exert pressure on the top of the foot with the other hand. This kneading motion produces a toning effect on the entire arch area.

Below: the kneading motion produces a toning effect on the entire arch area.

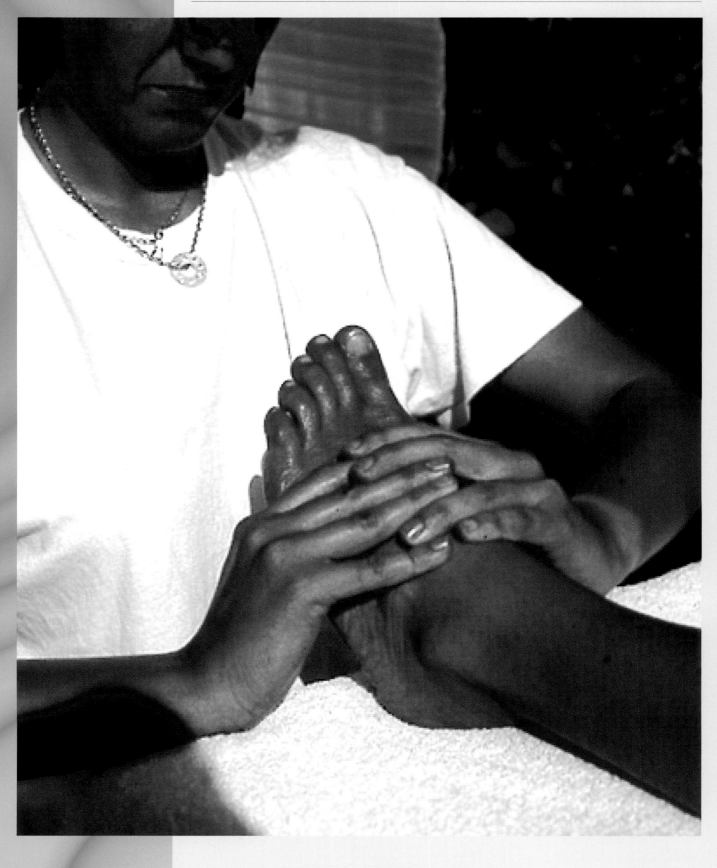

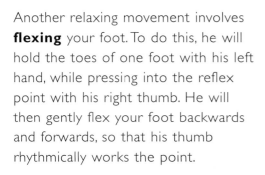

Another relaxing movement involves **flexing** your foot. To do this, he will hold the toes of one foot with his left hand, while pressing into the reflex point with his right thumb. He will then gently flex your foot backwards and forwards, so that his thumb rhythmically works the point.

Hooking out means that the therapist will apply pressure on the relevant point with his thumb. Next, he will draw back the thumb, making the shape of a fish hook on the sole of your foot.

It is only in the final stages of the treatment that your practitioner is likely to actually massage your feet. At this time, too, he may apply herbal cream or oil. Neither is used at the start of the treatment because the skin would then be too slippery to work on.

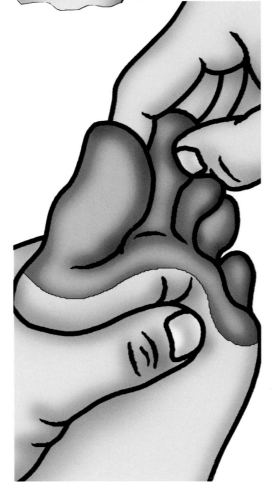

Above: another relaxing movement involves flexing your foot.

Left: the foot is flexed gently backwards and forwards.

Far left: it is only in the final stages of the treatment that your practitioner is likely to actually massage your feet.

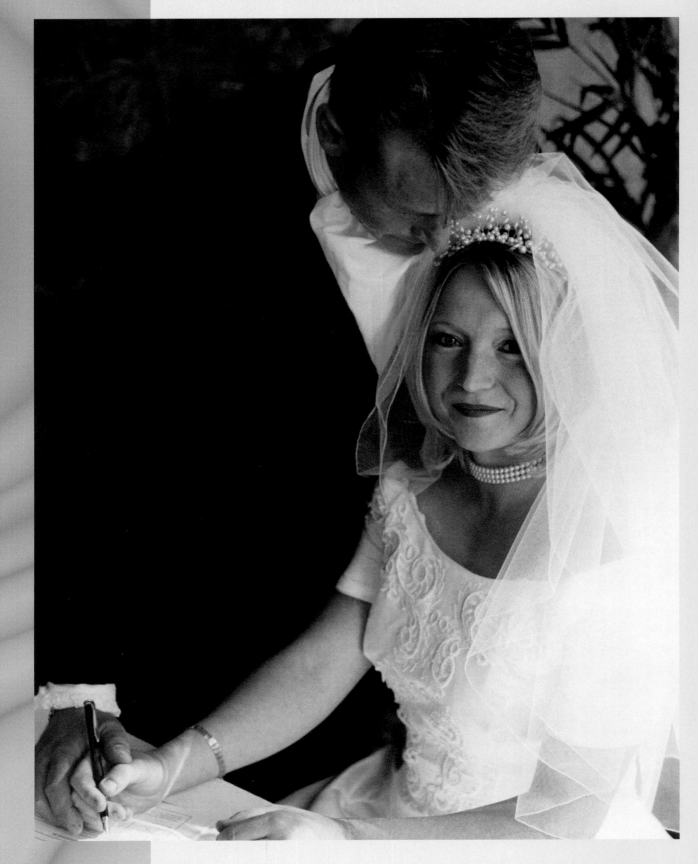

DEALING WITH STRESS

What does stress mean to you? In general, we use the term to indicate something we're not happy about. A traffic jam, too much work, a barking dog – all these and dozens of other daily events can produce the remark "It really stresses me out."

More positive happenings, too, can be stressful, though we don't always recognise this. Suppose you're planning to marry the love of your life and you've won the lottery. It seems that, for you, everything's coming up roses. But you are still in a stressful situation and clocking up 88 points on the Holmes-Rahe scale.

This is a system devised by two American doctors. It allocates a stress value to life events, according to the amount of physical and mental adjustment they need. The highest rating of 100 points goes to the death of husband or wife, the lowest (11 points) to a minor violation of the law. If you score 300 points or more in any one year, you are severely stressed. With 88 points from your marriage and your lottery win, you're more than a quarter of the way there.

It's obvious, then, that stress is a part of 21st-century living. How do we deal with it? The sad truth is that most of us don't – we simply become increasingly tense and bad-tempered. Only when our bodies begin to rebel and we find it difficult to cope with

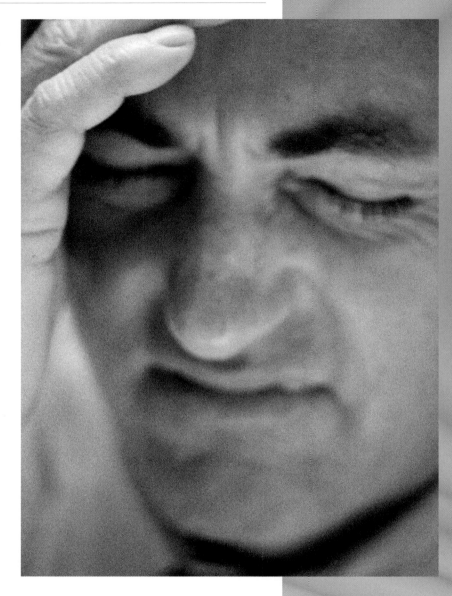

everyday life, do we attempt to remedy the situation.

If you are suffering from stress, your first step should be to examine your lifestyle. Are you eating a balanced diet, getting enough sleep and sufficient exercise? All these are important. You should also consider complementary therapies – and indulge yourself with a reflexology treatment every few weeks.

Far left: planning a wedding – a stressful situation and clocking up 88 points on the Holmes-Rahe scale.

Above: stress is part of 21st-century living.

WHOM REFLEXOLOGY CAN HELP

Both sexes and all ages can benefit from reflexology. In addition to inducing deep relaxation, it releases tension, stimulates the body parts where needed, and soothes physical and mental irritation.

Elderly people, in particular, often find it helps them to come to terms with modern living. They're constantly anxious – about the speed of life,

Below: reflexology is valuable to expectant mothers, helping to reduce the labour period.

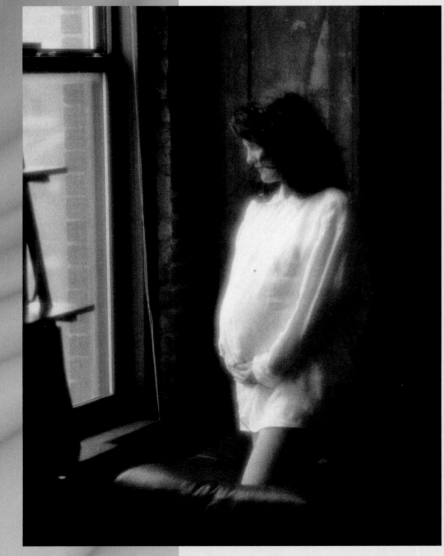

about today's high prices, about living alone, about their health and about dozens of things that the rest of us take for granted. All these stresses can be helped by reflexology treatment, as was proved in a Manchester hospital in 1990.

Some elderly patients, all suffering from stress, were divided into three groups. Group 1 received no treatment at all. Group 2 had an hour's counselling each day. Group 3 members were given an hour's reflexology treatment a day. At the end of eight days, all three groups were asked to assess their anxiety levels on a scale from 0 to 10. Group 1 recorded stress levels higher than before. Group 2 claimed that counselling had slightly eased their concerns. Group 3, who had received reflexology, showed a marked decrease in anxiety, in one case from eight stress points to one.

The treatment is valuable for expectant mothers, too. In 1995, a group of pregnant women were given a course of ten reflexology treatments in the hope that it would help them during childbirth. All were at least 20 weeks pregnant. When their babies were born, the women found that the time spent in labour was noticeably shorter than is usually the case.

Reflexology can help teenagers suffering from examination nerves, calm excitable children and soothe fractious babies. Children and babies are particularly receptive to the therapy.

Whatever our age or circumstances, reflexology treatment has been shown to be a valuable tool in bringing about the peaceful and harmonious life we all need. However, your first treatment should always be carried out by a qualified practitioner. Self-treatment, particularly by the elderly, pregnant women, diabetics and epileptics could cause problems which an experienced therapist would avoid. If you are receiving medical treatment, always let your doctor know if you intend to see a reflexologist.

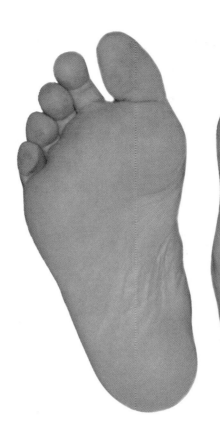

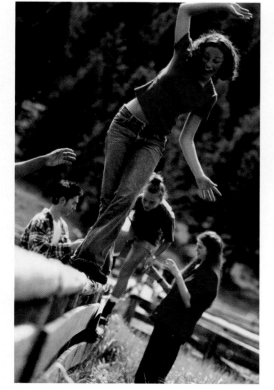

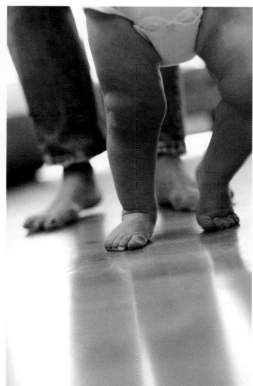

Left: reflexology can help teenagers suffering from examination nerves, calm excitable children and soothe fractious babies.

ALL ABOUT THE BODY SYSTEMS

Practitioners of complementary and orthodox medicine alike recognise that if the body is to be healthy, then it must be free from stress. When you have a reflexology treatment, you will swiftly appreciate that one of the most valuable benefits gained from it is relaxation, giving you renewed peace of mind.

Your physical body, too, needs to be released from tension. To achieve this complete harmony, all your body systems and reflexes need to be relaxed. This is where reflexology comes into its own. It can re-align the physical as well as the mental processes, and thus free the whole body system from stress. Let's consider where reflexology can help.

Right: the brain acts like an extremely complex computer that receives, sorts and interprets the messages delivered to it by nerves from every part of the body.

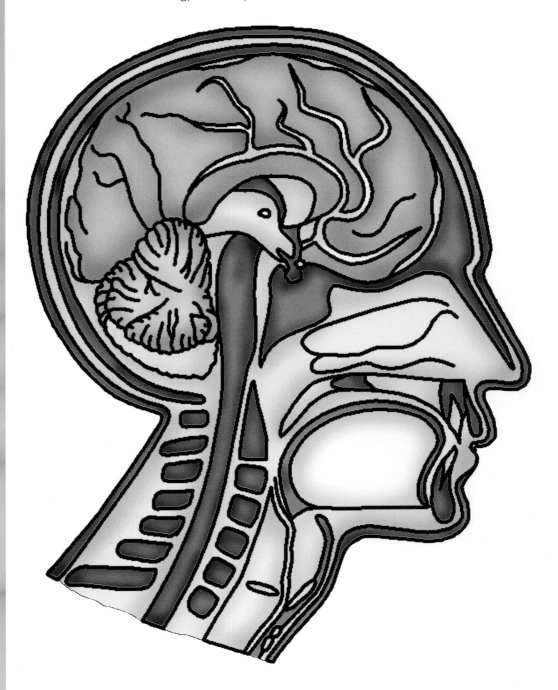

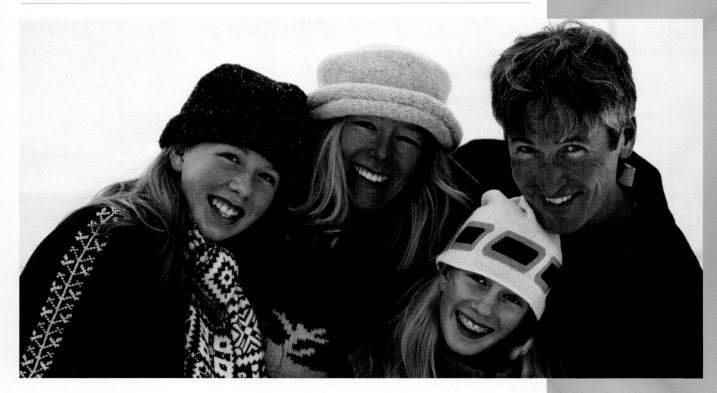

THE HEAD AREAS

The brain and the spinal cord together form your central nervous system (CNS) and are housed in the skull and the spine. The CNS controls all basic bodily functions, such as breathing, heart rate and body temperature. These are the systems over which we need have no control. Through evolution, we have handed over the operation of them to our brain. It acts like an extremely complex computer that receives, sorts and interprets the messages delivered to it by nerves from every part of the body. Then it reacts to these signals by sending out its own messages to the various parts of the body, telling them what to do.

For example, if you are cold, the temperature sensors in the skin send their message to the brain which reacts by sending messages to the muscles. These then start an involuntary movement that burns up energy and thus generates heat – it's called shivering.

Activities over which we do have control, including movement and speech, are also managed by the brain. Within the head, too, are some of our sensory areas which are associated with brain function, such as the nose, the palate, the eyes and ears. If the brain and CNS are not working correctly, then at least some of the associated functions will be impaired.

Above: if you are cold, the temperature sensors in the skin send their message to the brain.

Below: blood circulates the body 1,000 times per day or once every minute and a half.

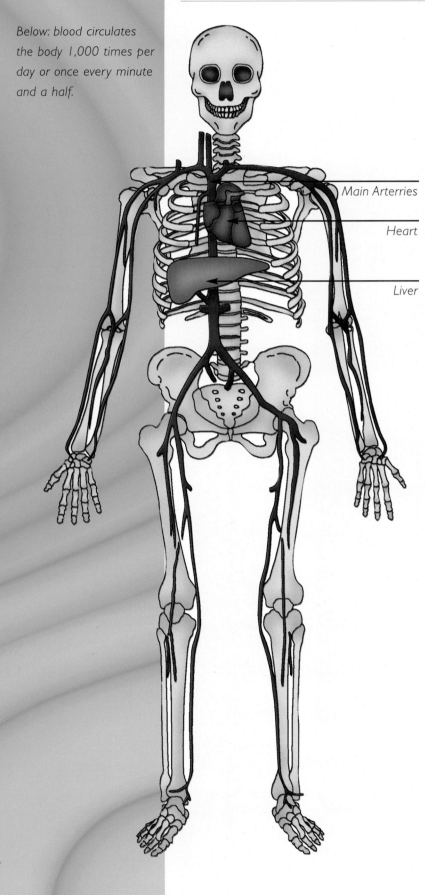

Main Arterries

Heart

Liver

THE CIRCULATORY SYSTEM

The circulatory (or cardiovascular) system is made up of the heart and thousands of blood vessels, permeating the whole body. Every cell of the body must have a continuous supply of oxygen-carrying blood in order for it to survive and function properly.

The heart beats unceasingly to keep pumping this essential blood to all parts of the body. In order to maintain this supply, it will continuously contract and expand something like 2,500 million times in an average lifetime. In everyday terms, this means that the heart pumps about 100,000 litres of blood through the system every 24 hours. The average body contains only six litres of blood. This means that the blood circulates the body 1,000 times per day or once every minute and a half. Should this blood supply be stopped for any reason. then life-giving oxygen will not reach the tissues and most will die very quickly.

THE DIGESTIVE SYSTEM

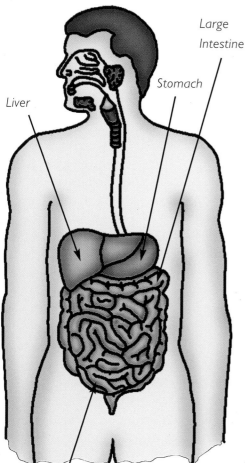

Liver

Large Intestine

Stomach

Small Intestine

The digestive system consists of the alimentary canal and various other associated organs. It goes from the mouth through some 35 feet of intestine to the rectum. Everything eaten and drunk passes through this system by waves of muscular contractions. As it goes, it is processed and absorbed, for building, repairing or nourishing the body. The remaining unusable portion of our food then moves on down through the digestive tract to the last part of the intestine, where water is removed before it is expelled from the body.

Left: the digestive system consists of the alimentary canal and various other associated organs.

Below: raw vegetables - nourishing the body

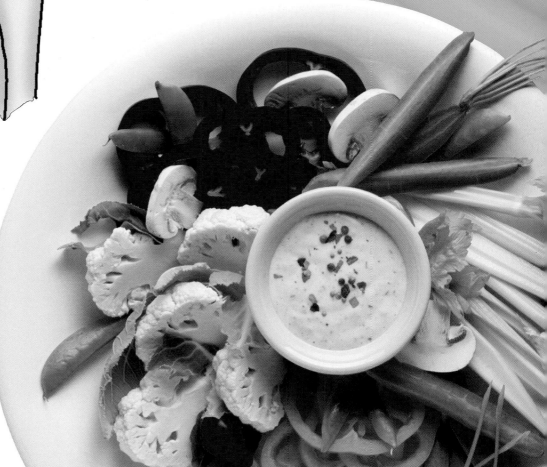

Right: to stimulate the endocrine system work on the reflex area of the pituitary gland contained in the brain reflex on the big toe. Then move on to the eye an ear reflexes on the toes of the same foot.

Below: lymph is vitally important to maintain the functioning of the immune system.

THE ENDOCRINE SYSTEM

The endocrine system consists of a collection of glands which secrete chemicals called hormones. These are essential to the normal functioning of the body. They include the pancreas, the adrenal cortex, the ovaries (in women), the testes (in men), the pituitary gland, the thyroid and parathyroid glands.

The hormones produced by these glands are responsible for many of the bodily functions over which we have no control. These include growth, metabolism, sexual development and function, and response to stress. Any increase or decrease in hormone production affects the process it controls and will inevitably lead to disease of one kind or another.

The most important lymphatic reflexes are found in the webs between the toes

To stimulate the endocrine system the reflex point is on the central point of the whorl on the big toe

Use either hand to support the foot

THE LYMPHATIC SYSTEM

The lymphatic system is closely connected to the blood circulatory system as it too carries fluid around the body. Like the blood system, it is circulatory. Lymph is a milky fluid made up of proteins, fats and white blood cells, and is carried in the lymph ducts. Functionally, it is also connected to the blood system, as its role is to collect any fluid that has escaped from the body tissues. Once collected, this is then returned to the blood system. At the same time, the lymphatic system collects and filters out any harmful bacteria found. Lymph is vitally important to maintain the functioning of the immune system.

THE MUSCULO-SKELETAL SYSTEM

Muscles are bundles of elongated cells that create movement by contracting and relaxing. Skeletal muscles (the body contains more than 600) are described as "voluntary". That is, they are under the voluntary control of the brain. Smooth muscles are concerned with movements of the internal organs as in digestion and in childbirth, and are not under our control. Cardiac muscles are found only in the heart. They contract about 100,000 times a day in order to maintain the flow of blood through the circulatory system.

Left: the body contains over 600 skeletal muscles which are described as 'voluntary' and are under the voluntary control of the brain.

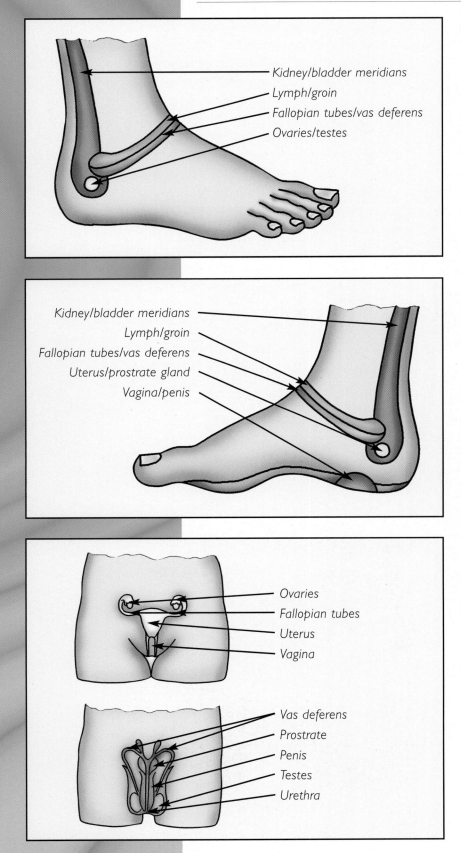

Kidney/bladder meridians
Lymph/groin
Fallopian tubes/vas deferens
Ovaries/testes

Kidney/bladder meridians
Lymph/groin
Fallopian tubes/vas deferens
Uterus/prostrate gland
Vagina/penis

Ovaries
Fallopian tubes
Uterus
Vagina

Vas deferens
Prostrate
Penis
Testes
Urethra

THE REPRODUCTIVE SYSTEM

In women, the reproductive system consists of the ovaries, fallopian tubes, uterus and vagina. The ovaries produce eggs once a month. These are either fertilised by the male sperm or are expelled as part of the menstrual cycle. They also produce the hormones that regulate this monthly cycle, plus secondary sexual characteristics such as facial hair and the depth of the voice. Any dysfunction of the ovaries will not only disrupt the normal cycle but will also produce an imbalance in many other parts of the body.

In men the reproductive system consists of the testes, prostate gland, vas deferens (the tube that carries the sperm from the testes) and the urethra (the tube that carries the sperm and urine down to the penis). In addition to sperm, the testes generate the male hormone testosterone that produces the male sexual characteristics. These include body bulk, facial and pubic hair, and depth of voice.

THE RESPIRATORY SYSTEM

The respiratory system is another term for the breathing apparatus. Its purpose is to extract oxygen from the air as you inhale, and pass it to the bloodstream. As you exhale, the waste product (carbon dioxide) carried by the blood is exchanged and expelled. The air inhaled passes through the nose or mouth to the lungs, and thus into the bloodstream. Inhalation and exhalation are facilitated by the chest muscles and the diaphragm.

A new baby takes about 40 breaths a minute, but in adults this speed is variable depending on whether the body is at rest and needs less oxygen, or active when more is needed. A resting adult breathes about 15 times a minute, but physical exertion can raise this rate to about 80 times a minute.

Far left: the reproductive system

Below: the respiratory system extracts oxygen from the air as you inhale, and passes it to the bloodstream.

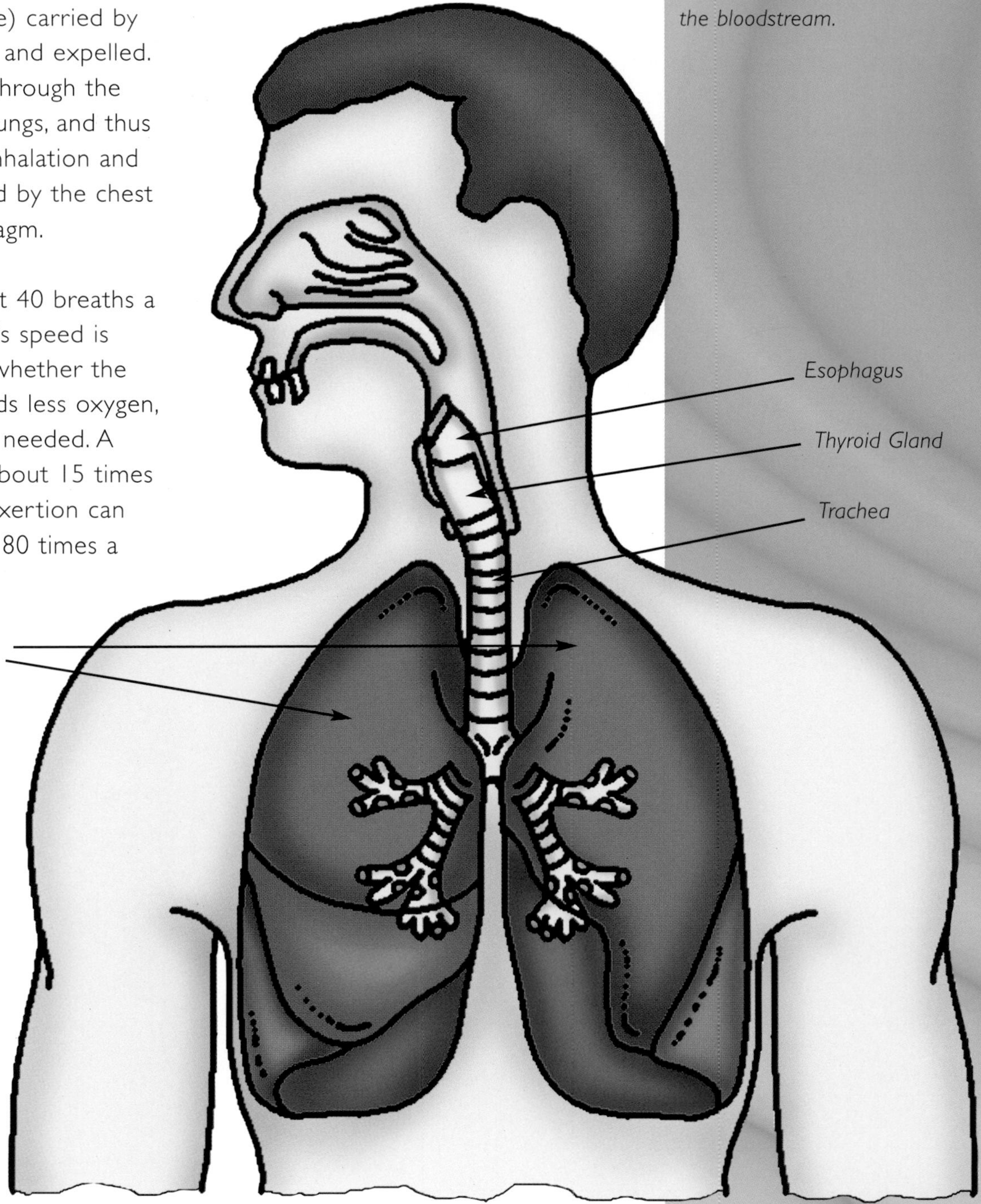

Esophagus

Thyroid Gland

Trachea

Lungs

Right: the urinary system carries waste matter, toxic materials and excess water away from the body.

The Urinary System

The urinary system is composed of two kidneys, two tubes called ureters, and the bladder. Its function is to carry waste matter, toxic materials and excess water away from the body.

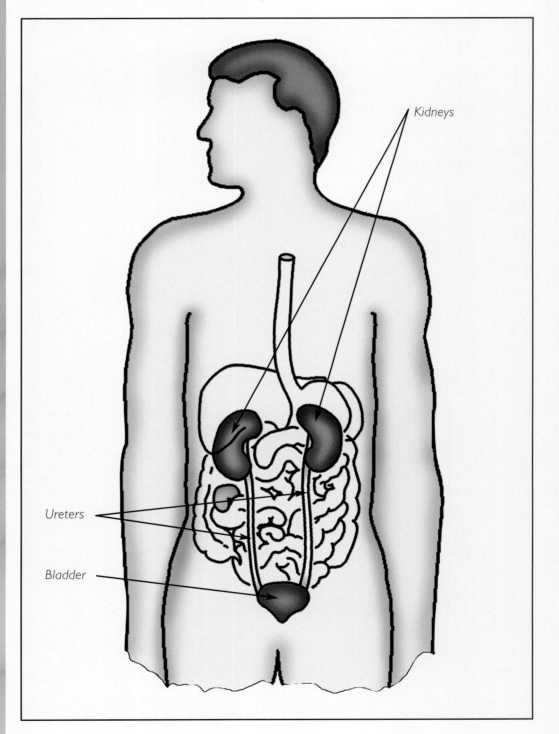

Kidneys

Ureters

Bladder

FINDING A REFLEXOLOGIST

It is illegal for anybody to claim to be a doctor if he is not medically qualified. Apart from that, it seems that in the UK anything goes. Unhappily, a number of unscrupulous people are trying to make a fast buck by jumping on the complementary therapy bandwagon.

So how can you be sure that your reflexologist is experienced and proficient? Contact one of the professional associations for reflexologists and ask for the names of members in your area. Be wary of advertisements in magazines and newspapers. Reflexologists are allowed to advertise, but cards in shop windows could indicate the amateur.

Don't be overly impressed, either, by a string of letters after his name. They could mean anything – or nothing. And be wary of correspondence courses. Some of these turn out "qualified" reflexologists, complete with certificates, after just half a dozen lessons. In reflexology, hands-on experience is essential.

There are many ways of becoming a qualified reflexologist. One man we know started out with a six-week introductory course at evening classes. Then he took the full works which involved studying for a year, using family and friends as guinea pigs. More courses followed – and now he has his own practice.

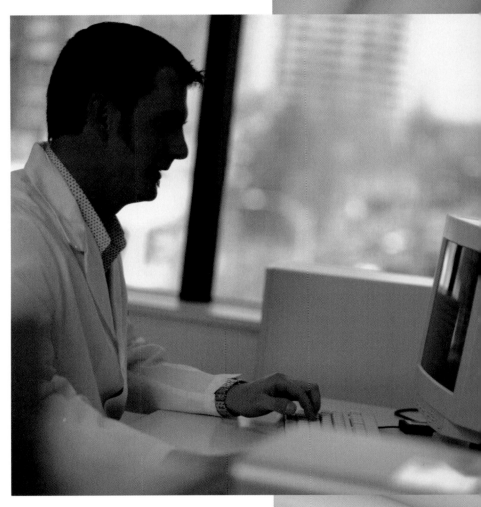

Below: one of the professional associations for reflexologists will have names of members in your area.

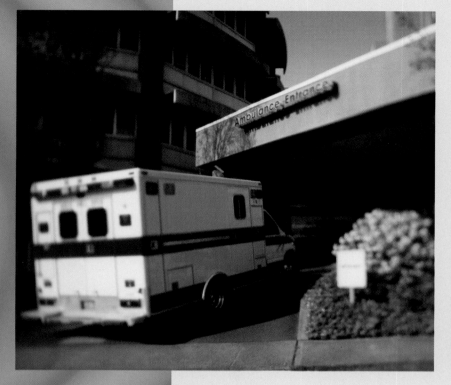

Above: nowadays, most towns boast at least one health centre..Some NHS hospitals have a reflexologist in attendance. This is unusual, but you may be lucky.

school where he trained is registered with the association.

Nowadays, most towns boast at least one health centre. It's safe to assume that any therapist practising there is beyond reproach – or you could even ask to be put in touch with satisfied clients. A health food shop may also be able to tell you about reflexologists in the area. Some NHS hospitals have a reflexologist in attendance. This is unusual, but you may be lucky.

In the end, though, it must be admitted that personal recommendation is by far the best way to find a reflexologist. If satisfied clients are prepared to recommend him, he must be doing something right.

If the practitioner claims that he is "fully trained", find out where he took his training. As with most other complementary therapies, there are a number of schools for reflexology. Sadly, not all of them have the same high standards. So, once you know the name of the training course your practitioner attended, you'd be well-advised to investigate the standing of that particular institution. Is it a reputable school? How long has it been established? How long does the training course take?

Most reflexologists are members of a professional body and will be happy to tell you which one. A swift phone call will enable you to check that he is a member and that the

There's one more question to ask. How much will the treatment cost? Don't expect to get good treatment at bargain prices. On the other hand, don't be conned into paying exorbitant amounts. Remember that you will need more than one visit and fees can mount up alarmingly.

TELL ME ABOUT A REFLEXOLOGY TREATMENT

Your first experience of reflexology should be relaxing and rewarding. To ensure this, you are advised to visit the practitioner's consulting room, rather than have him give the treatment in your own home. This will ensure that you are completely freed from the stress of everyday demands. No neighbours dropping in for coffee, no chores to do, no telephone calls, no family demands for attention.

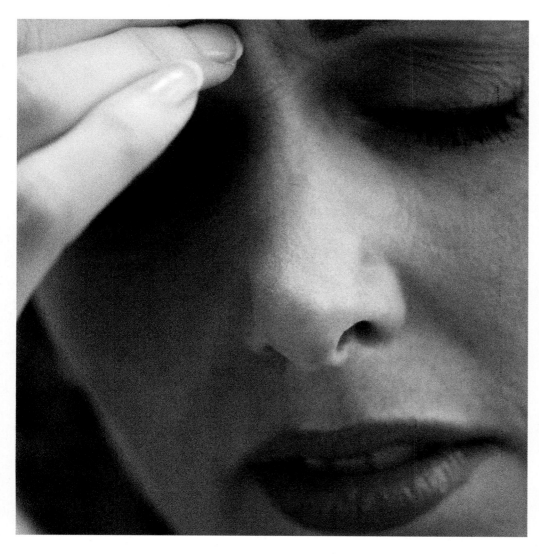

Left: for the duration of the consultation, attention will be focused completely on you - free from the stress of everyday demands

For the duration of the consultation, attention will be focused completely on you. These days, this is an unusual and delightful experience.

The consulting room will almost certainly be light and well ventilated, but comfortably warm. You may notice the fragrance of aromatherapy oils in the air and hear soft music in the background.

Right: the practitioner will want to record your medical history.

Below: a comprehensive account of past maladies and present difficulties will almost certainly give him some indication of how your current discomfort or dis-ease originated.

Before the treatment begins, the practitioner will want to record your medical history. Do be completely honest about this. Any problem, no matter how long ago it occurred, can be relevant. Tell him about any surgical procedures you have experienced, illnesses you have had, medication you are taking.

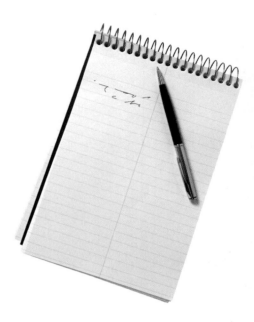

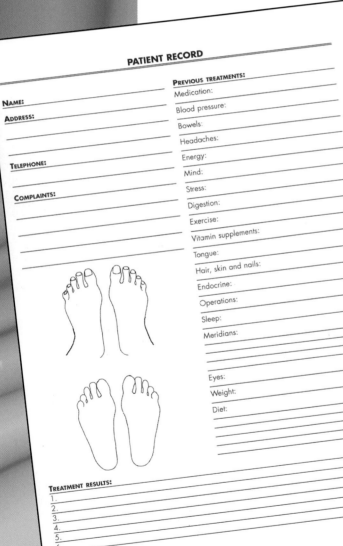

PATIENT RECORD

NAME:

ADDRESS:

TELEPHONE:

COMPLAINTS:

PREVIOUS TREATMENTS:

Medication:

Blood pressure:

Bowels:

Headaches:

Energy:

Mind:

Stress:

Digestion:

Exercise:

Vitamin supplements:

Tongue:

Hair, skin and nails:

Endocrine:

Operations:

Sleep:

Meridians:

Eyes:

Weight:

Diet:

TREATMENT RESULTS:
1.
2.
3.
4.
5.
6.

When these details have been recorded, he will ask about your present condition. You will be questioned about your bodily functions – bowels, bladder, digestion, menstrual and premenstrual problems – and about your lifestyle. He will enquire about your diet, how much exercise you take, whether you smoke or drink. Is your life stressful or relatively calm? Do you sleep well? Do you suffer from headaches?

Finally, he will want to know about the condition for which you are seeking treatment. Explain this as clearly as you can. A comprehensive account of past maladies and present difficulties will almost certainly give him some indication of how your current discomfort or dis-ease originated.

WRITE IT DOWN

If you feel at all nervous about this first treatment, perhaps it would be as well to write down the answers to these and similar questions before you keep your appointment. Write your own medical notes – a complete CV of your medical history. Such information really is important if the therapist is to get a clear idea of the state of your health. It would be a pity if your initial anxiety caused you to forget something.

Whilst this conversation has been taking place, you will probably have noticed a treatment couch or recliner chair in the room. You will now be invited to remove your shoes and hosiery and to take your place for treatment to begin.

Below: will probably have noticed a treatment couch or recliner chair in the room. You will now be invited to remove your shoes and hosiery and to take your place for treatment to begin.

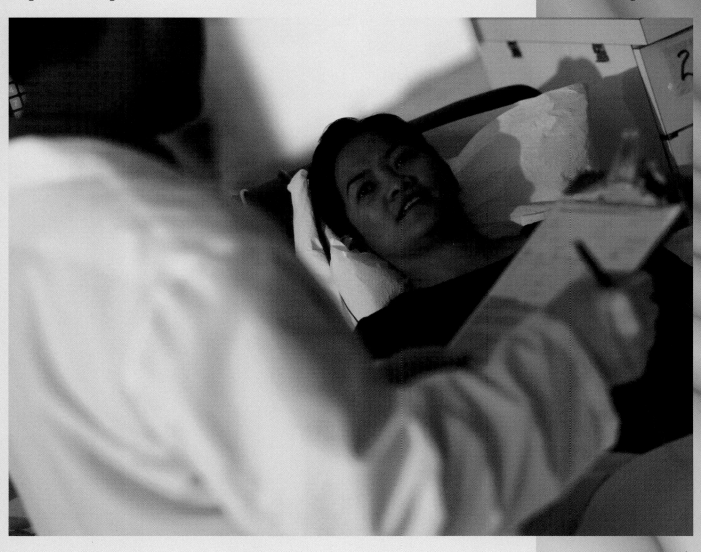

Below: some reflexologists start by sponging the feet with a mild disinfectant or witch hazel. The subsequent drying with a soft towel can begin the relaxation process.

This is when you may feel some embarrassment. Our poor neglected feet are rarely things of beauty. Displaying them to a complete stranger can be something of an ordeal. Don't worry. Your reflexologist has seen 'em all – and you will probably be reassured that your feet are less disgusting than you feared. Settle yourself comfortably on the couch and prepare to enjoy a pleasurable new experience.

Some reflexologists start by sponging the feet with a mild disinfectant or witch hazel. The subsequent drying with a soft towel can begin the relaxation process. A fine dusting of talcum powder comes next, to facilitate the movement of the practitioner's hands on your feet.

Treatment usually begins with massage, employing a gentle stroking movement. This is followed by a close examination of your feet, from which the practitioner will gain a clear picture of your problems. You have probably never noticed the different colours of the skin on your feet. Look now and you will see that they exist. To the practitioner, these can give indications of imbalance. Different colours will indicate different conditions to him.

This is followed by a much firmer massage of the reflex areas. You may notice that the practitioner uses his thumb to apply pressure to the reflex points. Each point is about the size of a pinhead and there are dozens of them in each area, so precision is vital.

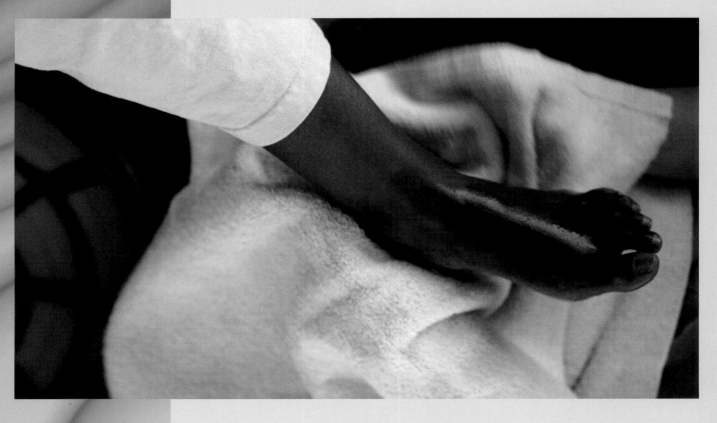

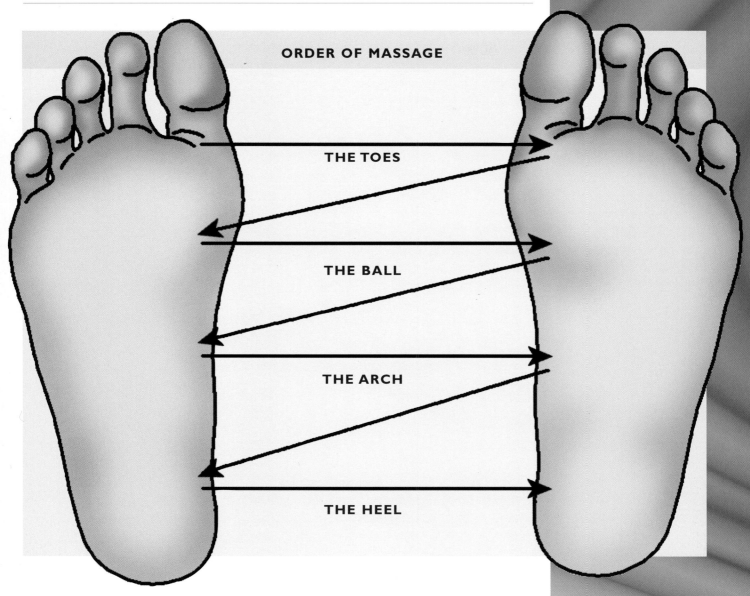

ORDER OF MASSAGE

THE TOES

THE BALL

THE ARCH

THE HEEL

Usually, your right sole will be treated first, working from the tips of your toes down to the heel. This is followed by massage of the top and sides of the foot, before repeating the procedure on the left foot. However, some practitioners prefer to alternate – working on the toes of the right foot, then the toes of the left, and so on.

Reflexology should not be painful. If you do experience pain in any particular area, this indicates some form of blockage in the corresponding part of the body. The tender area will then require extra attention to clear the congestion.

Above: usually, your right sole will be treated first, working from the tips of your toes down to the heel.

HOW WILL I FEEL AFTER TREATMENT?

Although most people enjoy reflexology, post-treatment reactions can vary. It is quite normal to experience some tingling in your arms and legs, but this is not unpleasant. You may be so completely relaxed that you could happily fall asleep on the couch or you could feel revitalised and full of energy.

For the first hour or so after receiving reflexology, try to take things quietly. Relax. Resist any urge to "get up and go", no matter how energetic you feel.

Above: the treatment is usually completed within an hour

Right: you may be so completely relaxed that you could happily fall asleep on the couch or you could feel revitalised and full of energy.

HOW LONG DOES IT TAKE?

The treatment is usually completed within an hour, though a first consultation often takes longer because the therapist needs to discuss your medical history. Depending on the condition being treated, subsequent treatments could last for only 30/40 minutes. Rely on your practitioner to recognise your needs. Too much treatment can be over-stimulating. On the other hand, a session that is too brief will not provide sufficient stimulation for the body to benefit.

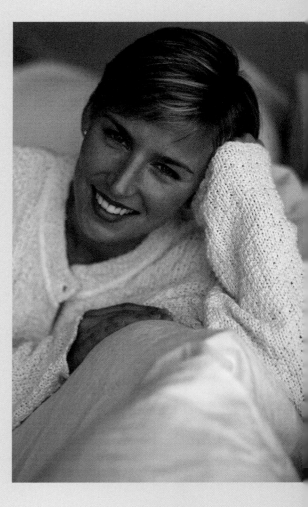

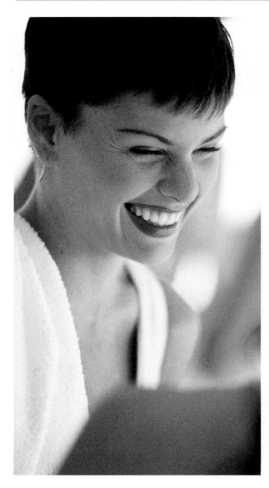

Do be aware that a "healing crisis" may occur at some stage, sometimes after the first treatment. This is not nearly as ominous as it sounds. Don't be alarmed if you develop what appears to be a heavy head cold, break out in a skin rash, feel slightly giddy or extremely tired. These and other minor ailments are part of the healing process. They show that you are responding to treatment and there is no need to worry about them. Increasing your liquid intake will help to flush the toxins out of your system. Extra rest may help, too. In any case, these adverse reactions will swiftly pass. Consult your reflexologist if you are at all concerned, but do resist the temptation to treat yourself with over-the-counter drugs.

Not everybody experiences a healing crisis. Two of the most immediate results of the first consultation are usually a better sleeping pattern and a more easy-going frame-of-mind. Subsequent treatments can only increase the feeling of well-being and calm. So gradually that you may not even notice it at first, your problems will fade and your whole approach to life will be more laid-back.

Above right; a better sleeping pattern.

Above left: an increased feeling of well-being and calm.

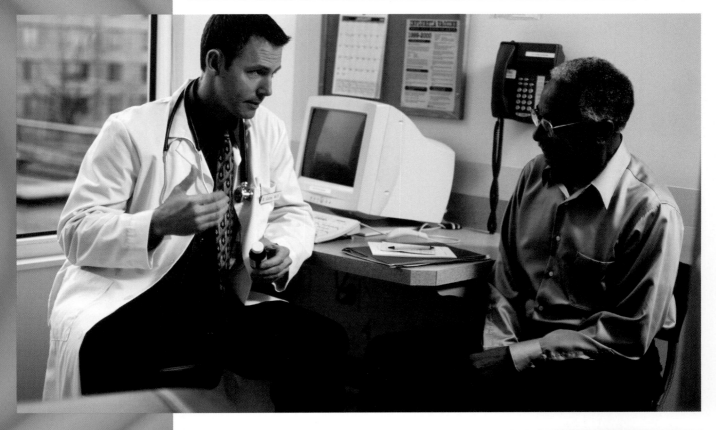

Above: most people recognise a marked improvement in their condition by the time they have visited the reflexologist three times.

Right: perhaps another form of complementary therapy would suit you better.

How Often do I Need Treatment?

Frequency of treatment depends on a number of factors. Most people recognise a marked improvement in their condition by the time they have visited the reflexologist three times. In the unlikely event that there is no improvement at all, you should begin to wonder if your particular problem is going to be responsive to the treatment. Discuss this with your therapist. Perhaps another form of complementary therapy would suit you better.

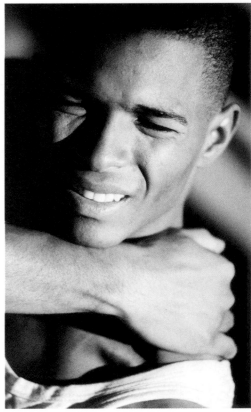

If your problems are long-standing, you may need extra sessions to solve them. Similarly, if you have been taking medication, your condition may appear to worsen slightly at first because the symptoms have been suppressed by drugs. Even if your problems disappear after the initial consultation, you would be well advised to continue with a short course of treatment to ensure that this happy state is maintained.

When any part of the body has been disturbed, it takes time to restore the balance. Most reflexologists advise a course of eight weekly treatments. It could be a good idea, too, to have a "topping up" session occasionally to maintain your equilibrium.

Again – take your therapist's advice.

Below:take your therapist's advice.

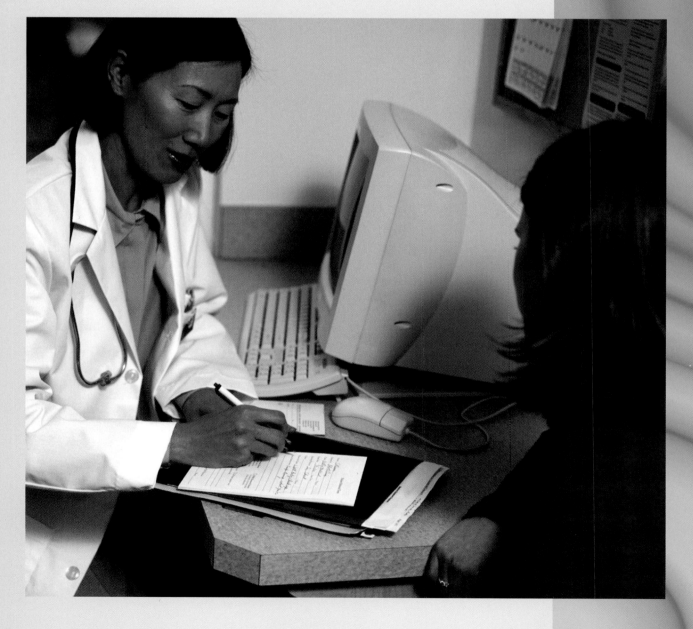

WHAT CAN I EXPECT FROM MY REFLEXOLOGIST?

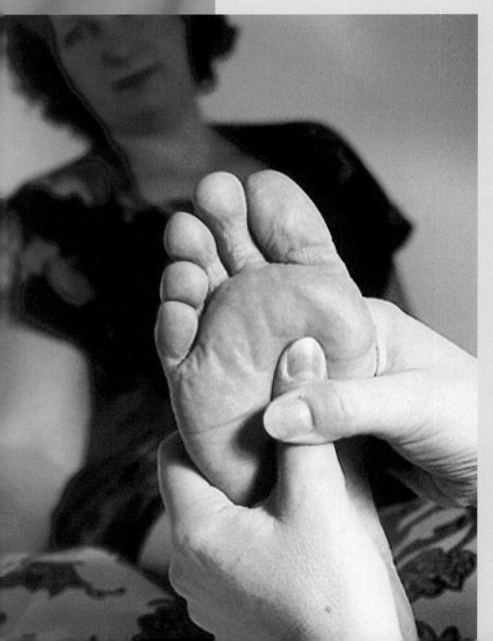

Below: you should feel completely at ease and perfectly safe in your therapist's company. If there is anything at all about the reflexologist or his surroundings that makes you feel uneasy, go elsewhere.

All good reflexologists regard themselves as professionals, That being so, you have a right to expect only the highest standards in every aspect of your treatment.

The consulting room should be absolutely clean, tidy and as quiet as possible. Some practitioners do work from home, but most set aside a room for the purpose. It's not a good idea to recline on the family sofa while receiving treatment.

The therapist's attitude should be calm and reassuring. Having written down your medical history, he should then be prepared to give you a simple explanation of the treatment he is going to give you. This is the time to ask questions about anything which worries or puzzles you.

He should be friendly, but not familiar. Some reflexologists prefer to work in silence, so that their full attention is on the treatment they are giving. Others feel that a gentle flow of conversation relaxes their patients.

The practitioner's appearance should be immaculate. A white coat is not mandatory, and some therapists prefer a more casual style of clothing. Whatever is worn, though, the clothing should be spotless as should the hands and nails.

And finally – you should feel completely at ease and perfectly safe in your therapist's company. If there is anything at all about the reflexologist or his surroundings that makes you feel uneasy, go elsewhere. Even if the problem is merely a personality clash, it's best to find a practitioner with whom you feel completely relaxed.

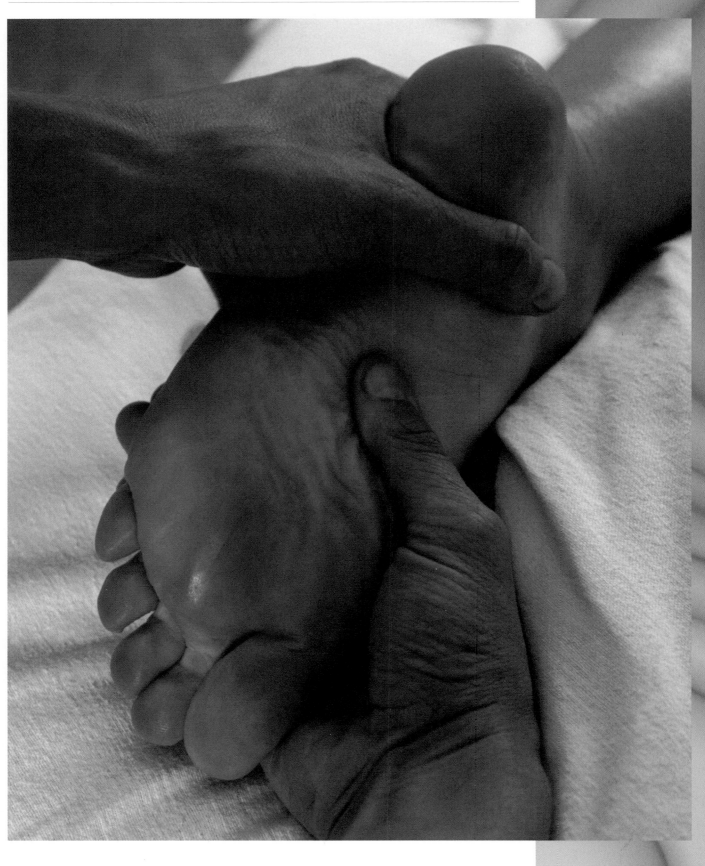

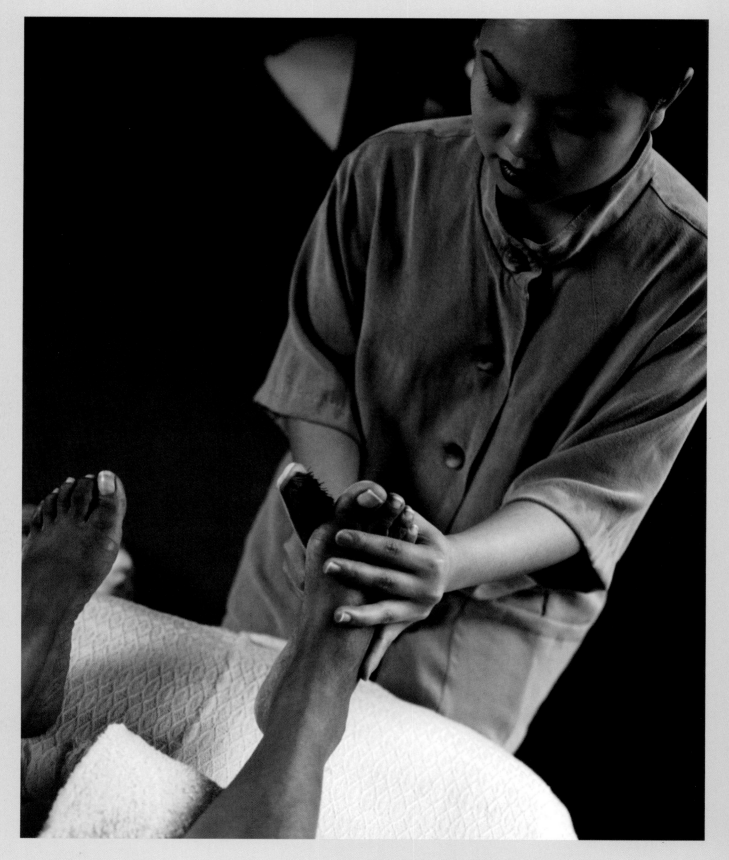

DIY REFLEXOLOGY

It's not possible to give yourself a complete reflexology treatment. You won't be able to reach all the reflex points. Additionally, most of us would find it difficult to sit cross-legged for an hour, on a bed or on the floor.

The alternative of sitting on a chair with one foot raised on to the opposite knee is equally uncomfortable.

DIY reflexology can never be as beneficial as treatment from a qualified practitioner. Even so, it will tide you over until you can make an appointment for a professional consultation.

TREATING YOURSELF

You must first consider exactly why you need to treat yourself. Do you have particular symptoms you want to relieve? Then it may be as well to work specifically on those reflexes which you know are imbalanced. You don't need professional training to do this. Once you've decided on the problem you most want to deal with, you need to check which reflexes are involved. The chart on page 25 will help you to do this. Once you are clear in your mind about which reflex areas need attention, you're ready to start. So how do you go about this?

Avoid constricting clothing in favour of something loose and comfortable. Prepare the room, ensuring that it is warm but not stuffy. Disconnect the phone. Put the cat out. If you fancy lighting a scented candle or playing some soothing music, do it now.

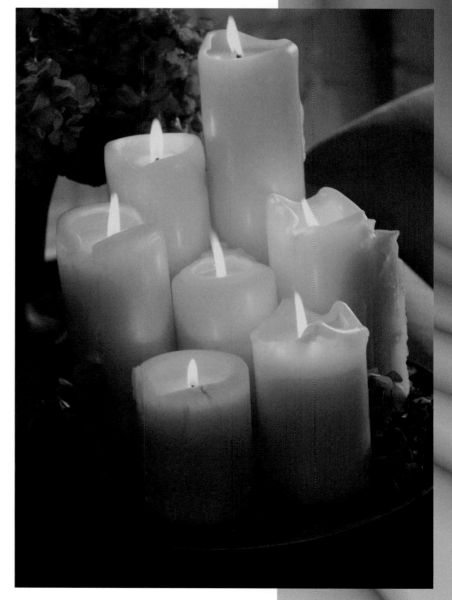

Far leftt: DIY reflexology can never be as beneficial as treatment from a qualified practitioner.

Below: light a scented candle or play some soothing music to create a relaxing atmosphere.

Before you start the session, have a few minutes of complete relaxation. Close your eyes. Breathe slowly and deeply. Try to visualise clearly exactly how you are going to give the treatment. This is important. You don't want to try to read instructions from a book at the same time that you're following them.

When you are ready to begin, make yourself as comfortable as possible. It's irritating if you have to break off mid-treatment to push cushions behind your back.

Let us suppose you have a bit of a headache and would like to get rid of it. This condition is often the result of a build-up of tension. That being so, you should concentrate your efforts on the reflex points corresponding to the neck. These are to be found at the tips of the big toes, so this is the area in which you should apply gentle pressure. The operative word here is "gentle".

Next turn your attention to the head reflex itself. You'll find this on the pads of the big toes. Again – easy does it. Don't press too hard or for longer than one or two seconds.

This type of treatment is simple and brief, but is likely to produce highly satisfactory results. When you've finished, lie back and relax for a quarter of an hour – and don't be surprised if you fall asleep.

TWIDDLE YOUR TOES

Having tried one form of self-treatment, you may be interested in trying something else. This focuses on the whole foot, not just the two big toes. With this method, you don't need to concentrate on specific reflexes. Simply stroking your feet and wriggling your toes can be highly effective. Play "this little piggy went to market" any time you feel in need of relaxation/ refreshment.

Below: before you start the session, have a few minutes of complete relaxation.

Far right: simply stroking your feet and wriggling your toes can be highly effective.

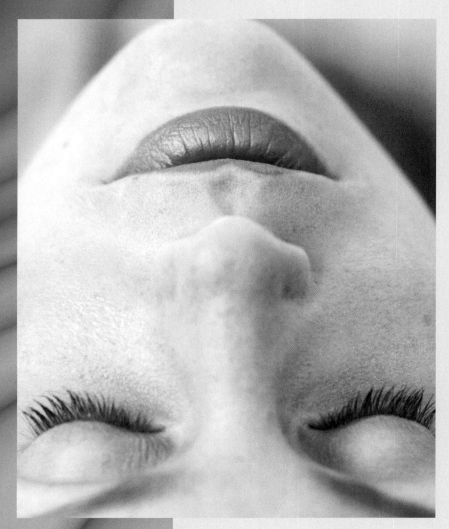

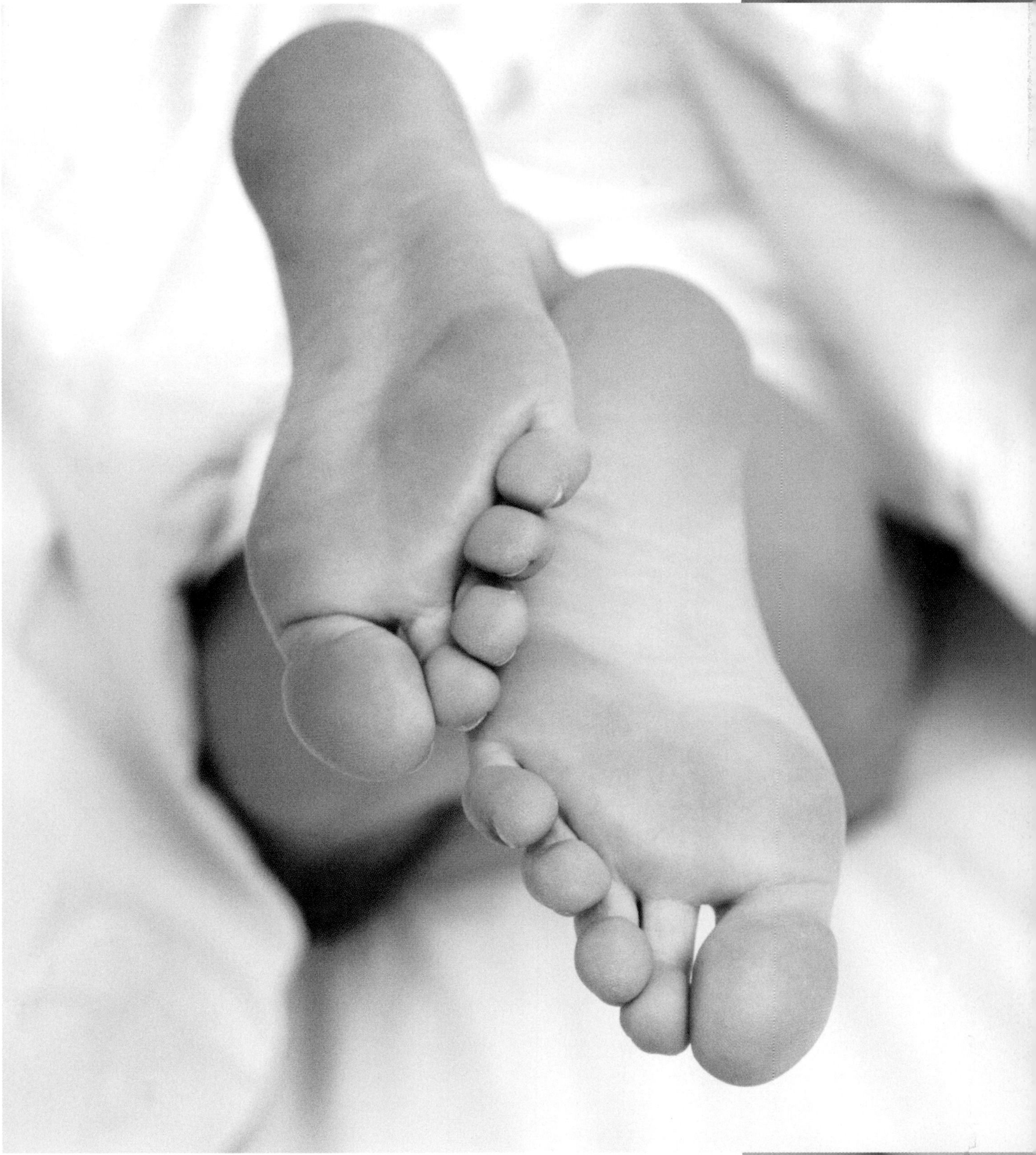

HAND REFLEXOLOGY

Most people equate reflexology with the feet, but it can work equally well on your hands. Like the feet, the hands carry reflex areas corresponding to all parts of the body.

You will usually find that your hands are less sensitive than your feet, partly because hands are constantly in use while feet are protected by footwear. But because the hand is smaller than the foot, it can be more difficult to locate the reflex points. Perhaps this is the reason most reflexologists prefer to work on the feet. In America, though, it is usual to work both hands and feet during a treatment.

In self-treatment, you will find that working on the hands is more simple than on the feet, because they are easier to reach. The reflex areas are exactly the same as those in the feet and respond in precisely the same fashion.

Another advantage in using the hands for self-treatment is that this can be undertaken almost anywhere at any time. You can give yourself a treatment while you're waiting for a bus, watching television – even during a lecture or at a meeting. The great advantage is that nobody else will be aware of what you are doing.

Hand reflexology is particularly useful for dealing with anxiety, menstrual pain or headaches, and can sometimes help fertility problems (though this is best left to the professionals.)

If you suffer from osteoporosis or thrombosis or if you are running a high temperature, you must not use hand reflexology.

Right: you will usually find that your hands are less sensitive than your feet, partly because hands are constantly in use

REFLEX POINTS OF THE HAND

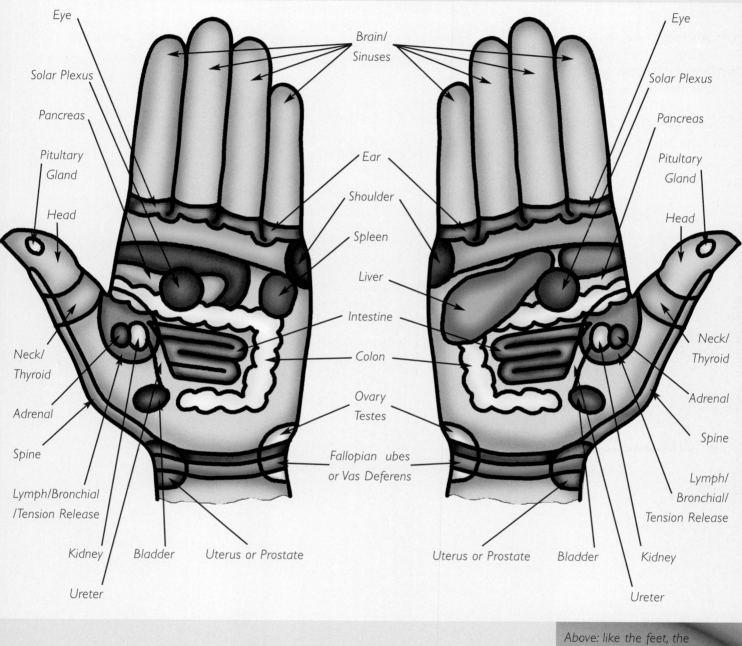

Eye
Solar Plexus
Pancreas
Pitultary Gland
Head
Neck/Thyroid
Adrenal
Spine
Lymph/Bronchial /Tension Release
Kidney
Ureter
Bladder
Uterus or Prostate

Brain/ Sinuses
Ear
Shoulder
Spleen
Liver
Intestine
Colon
Ovary Testes
Fallopian ubes or Vas Deferens

Eye
Solar Plexus
Pancreas
Pitultary Gland
Head
Neck/ Thyroid
Adrenal
Spine
Lymph/ Bronchial/ Tension Release
Uterus or Prostate
Bladder
Kidney
Ureter

Above: like the feet, the hands carry reflex areas corresponding to all parts of the body.

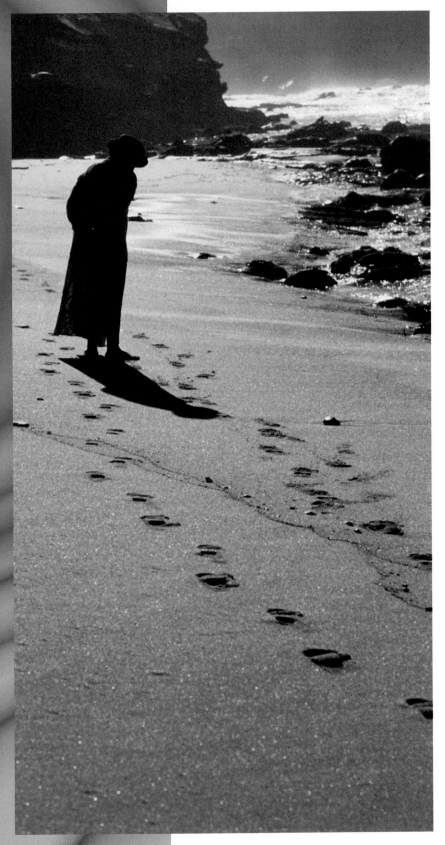

What Else You can Do

If you are wary of attempting reflexology on yourself or if you don't have time to spare for any of these treatments, you can still refresh your feet and release any tension you are feeling. Try walking barefoot as often as you can. Walking on grass or a sandy beach or paddling in the sea are great experiences – but be sure there's no risk of injuring your feet on broken glass or stones.

Lacking such ideal conditions, make a habit of walking barefoot at home. When you're sitting down, try rolling a golf ball or a small bottle between your foot and the floor. Any form of foot exercise can be useful and is almost guaranteed to lift your spirits.

CARING FOR YOUR FEET

Do you know how far you walk in a day? Probably not, but it is estimated that the average person clocks up about 1,000 miles a year. That's less than three miles a day, but it means that by the time you reach your 70th birthday, your poor feet will have supported your full weight – plus anything else you may be carrying – for at least 70,000 miles. How many pairs of shoes would you expect to get through in that time?

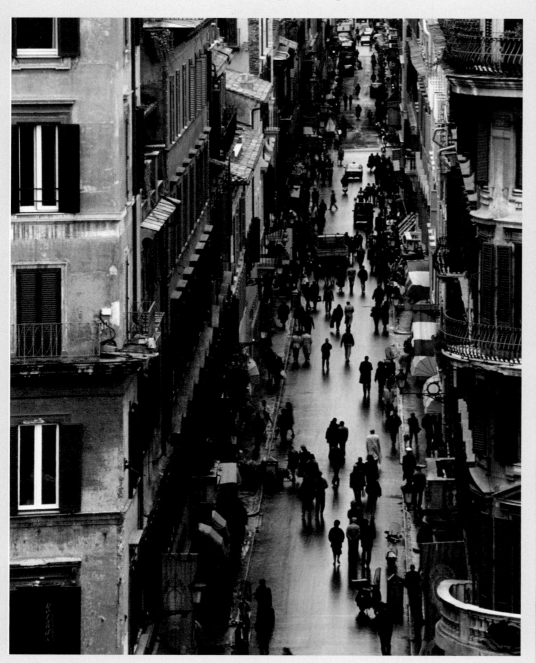

Far left: walking on grass or a sandy beach or paddling in the sea are great experiences.

Left: the average person clocks up about 1,000 miles a year.

When we buy a new pair of shoes, we take care of them. We put them on trees when they're not in use and try to maintain their pristine appearance. When they start to get shabby, we buy new laces to spruce them up, polish them regularly, and get them mended. Eventually they wear out and we dispose of them.

When shoes wear out, they can be replaced with new ones. Feet can't. Shoes can be mended, given new soles and heels. Feet can't.

Considering we "wear" the same pair of feet for the whole of our lives, it's surprising that we don't give them the same – or more – attention that we give to our shoes. Caring for your feet is a simple affair and doesn't take long. The result will be well worth the time and effort involved. Not only will your feet look and feel better – your general health will also benefit.

Far left: when shoes wear out, they can be replaced with new ones. Feet can't.

Below: when shoes start to get shabby, we get them mended.

Below left: the warmth and moisture from your feet provides a perfect breeding ground for bacteria.

Below right: wash them every day, probably when you have a bath – but do you take particular care with drying them?

FOOT HYGIENE

There's more to foot hygiene than just keeping your feet clean. Of course you wash them every day, probably when you have a bath – but do you take particular care with drying them? When you consider that your feet sweat out about a cupful of moisture every day, it makes sense to ensure that they're really dry after you've washed them.

The warmth and moisture from your feet provides a perfect breeding ground for bacteria. This can result in athlete's foot and all sorts of fungal infections, not to mention bromhidrosis – that's the polite term for smelly feet. In hot weather, it's a good idea to hold your feet under running water several times a day. This keeps them cool, comfortable and inoffensive.

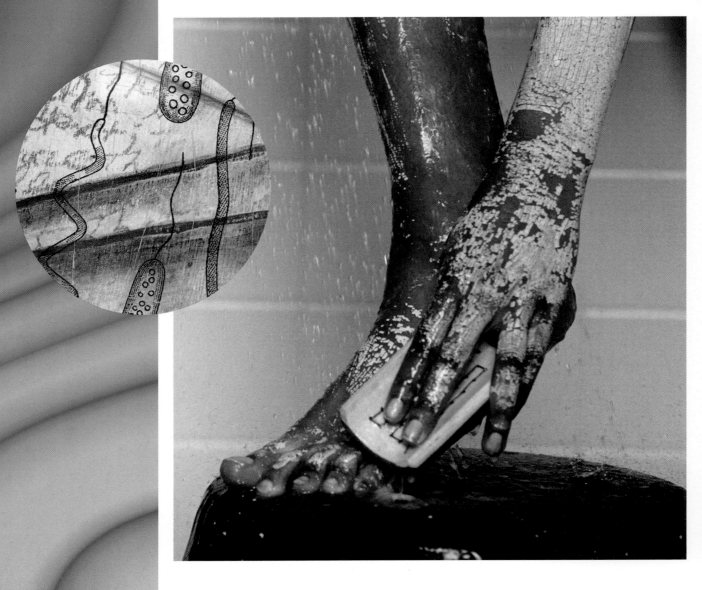

FOOTWEAR

Try always to wear leather shoes, so that your feet can breathe. If you prefer trainers, be prepared to invest in expensive leather ones rather than cheap plastic. Remember, too, that allowing your children to wear colourful "jelly" footwear could well result in foot problems by the time they reach their teens, plus sinus troubles, a tendency to head colds and various other irritations or dis-eases.

Ensure that your shoes (and socks or tights) are a perfect fit. Socks should be made from natural fibres such as wool or cotton. Change them every day – more often in hot weather. If they shrink when washed, throw them out. Socks that are too small are as constricting – and therefore as damaging – as tight shoes.

Flat-heeled, soft leather sandals are the best possible type of footwear, but obviously it's not always acceptable to wear them. If high heels are essential for specially smart occasions, compensate by replacing them with flatties as soon as you get home.

Above: try always to wear leather shoes, so that your feet can breathe. If you prefer trainers, be prepared to invest in expensive leather ones rather than cheap plastic.

Right: Slippers are not glamorous, but they will protect your feet against sudden temperature changes.

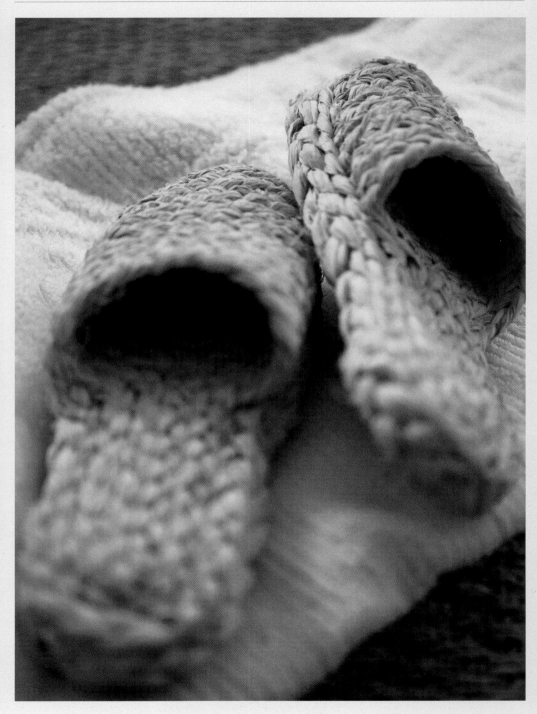

Sudden temperature changes are bad for your feet. Running barefoot from the warmth of a carpeted bedroom to the chill of a tiled bathroom floor gives your reflexes a nasty shock, and can well affect corresponding body parts. Don't disdain a pair of slippers. They're certainly not glamorous, but they're soft and comfortable and will protect your feet.

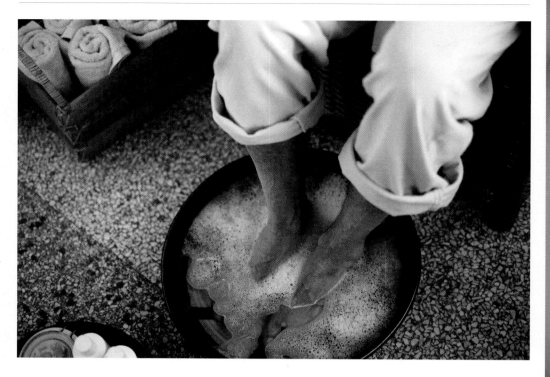

Left: invest in a foot bath.
A washing-up bowl works
just as well, but there's
something luxurious
about dunking your feet
in a utensil reserved for
the purpose.

TLC FOR FEET

If you've neglected your feet for years, a visit to a chiropodist is a good idea. Chiropody is a soothing experience and, if you watch carefully, you'll learn a lot from just one session. If you have painful problems like corns or ingrowing toenails, you'll probably need more than one treatment. Usually, though, it's easy to care for your own feet and just one visit to a chiropodist gets you off to a good start.

First – invest in a foot bath. A washing-up bowl works just as well, but there's something luxurious about dunking your feet in a utensil reserved for the purpose. Have the water as hot as you can bear, but be careful not to scald your feet. Add a few herbs – lavender or marjoram – or a couple of drops of aromatherapy oil, and immerse your feet for no more than five minutes.

Dry them carefully, then gently use a pumice stone on any hard skin. Don't overdo it. It may take several attempts to dispose of callouses that have built up over a long period.

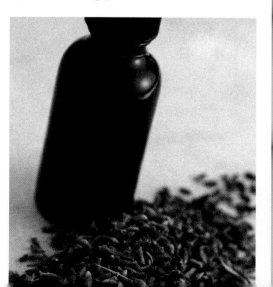

Far right: chiropody is a soothing experience and, if you watch carefully, you'll learn a lot from just one session. If you have painful problems like corns or ingrowing toenails, you'll probably need more than one treatment.

Below: footcare utensils

Use clippers or sharp scissors to trim your toenails. Always cut the nails straight across, not curved down at the sides. This can lead to ingrowing toenails. Apply a little oil to your cuticles to keep them supple, but never be tempted to cut them back.

And that's all you need to do for a home pedicure. Simple, isn't it?

If you're feeling really self-indulgent, why not massage your feet with sweet smelling oil or a herbal foot cream? You can also invest in some aids to help you exercise your feet. Look around in your local branch of Boots or any other large chemist. You'll find lots of foot-care gadgets and most of them are effective.

TLC for feet can be fun.

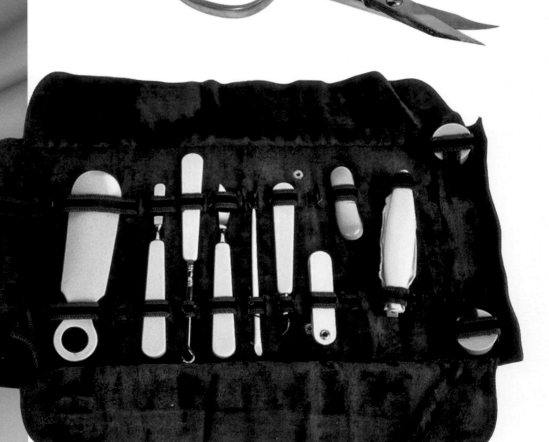

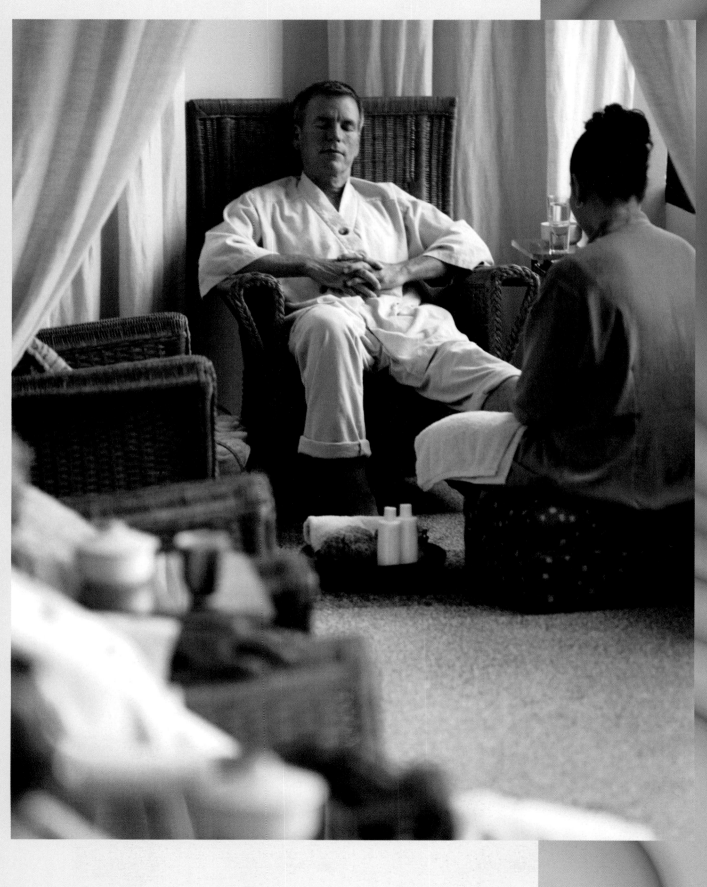

*Below: more and more
people are turning to
complementary/alternative
medicine.*

REFLEXOLOGY TODAY

The past two decades have seen a surge of interest in what is known as the holistic approach. Medical specialists are no longer regarded as minor gods who know everything. Instead, most people recognise that bodily dis-ease cannot be treated in isolation. Body, mind and spirit are inextricably interwoven and treatment must involve all three.

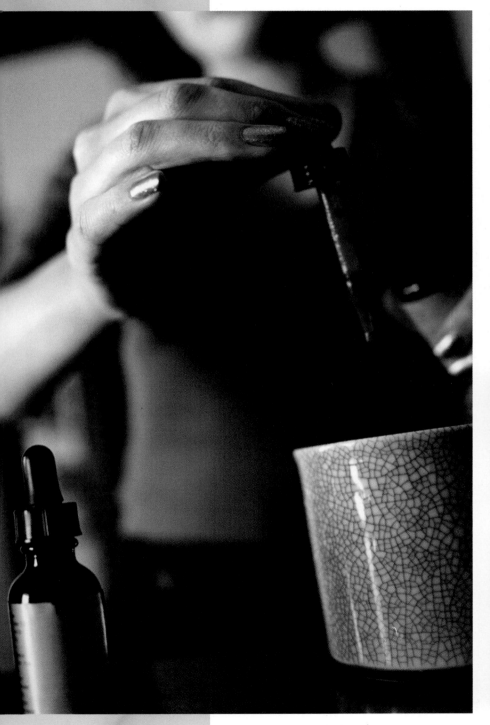

As a result of this realisation, more and more people are turning to complementary/alternative medicine. We are accepting responsibility for our own well-being but, because few of us are medical experts, we are looking to ancient remedies for help.

Reflexology is one such therapy. It dates back thousands of years, but since its introduction to the UK in the 1960s new methods have developed alongside the more traditional ones. Some of these advances include complementary therapies as ancient as reflexology itself. Others involve more modern techniques.

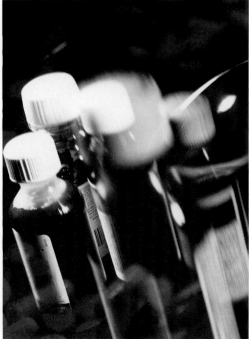

VACUFLEX REFLEXOLOGY

This system is thought to have originated in Denmark in the 1960s. It combines three types of treatments – reflexology, acupressure and the little-known but ancient practice called cupping.

Originally, the cups were heated, so as to expand the air inside, before being applied to the body. As the air cooled, it contracted and formed a partial vacuum, drawing the flesh into the cup and literally sucking out any poison that might be present. Nowadays, a vacuum pump is used for the same purpose.

The first "cups" were made from animal horns. Others, discovered in Mesopotamia, were made from fired clay and in Greece bronze was used. Porcelain, brass and glass cups have also been found on archeological sites. Less romantically, 21st-century VacuFlex cups are referred to as "pads" and are made of silicone.

Below: the ancient practice of cupping.

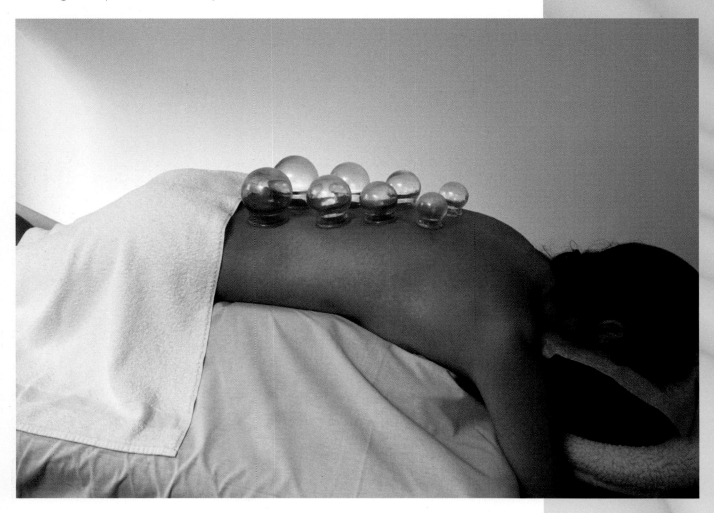

When you go for a VacuFlex treatment your feet will be encased in what can only be described as huge felt space-boots. These are connected to a a vacuum pump that suctions the air from all round your feet. The resulting air pressure presses the boot against every part of each foot. It's a tremendously relaxing process, which clears any blockages and aids circulation.

The boots are worn for only ten minutes. When they are removed, a map of colours is revealed on your feet. These colours are visible for only about 15 seconds. They show the therapist exactly where further normal reflexology treatment is needed and give an accurate indication of the severity of the problem.

Blue or blue/black patches show where the body is under acute stress. Red reveals acid deposits and suggest that there are high sugar levels in the body. White indicates long-standing congestion. Yellow around the lung reflex could suggest asthma or similar problems.

The system works well for children. The idea of wearing space-boots which produce glorious technicolour patterns on their feet holds a strong appeal for most youngsters.

VacuFlex reflexology is claimed to be successful with such widely varying problems as arthritis, migraine, insomnia and eczema. It's also particularly good at dealing with back pain.

Below: VacuFlex boots are connected to a a vacuum pump that suctions the air from all round your feet.

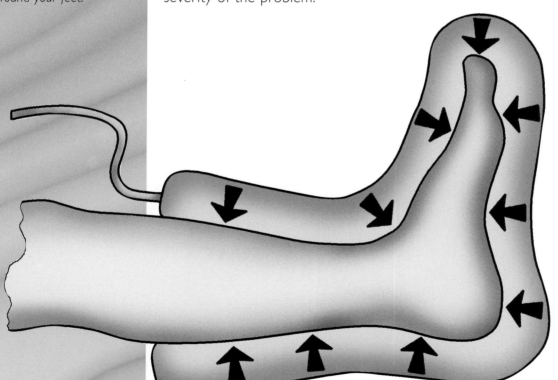

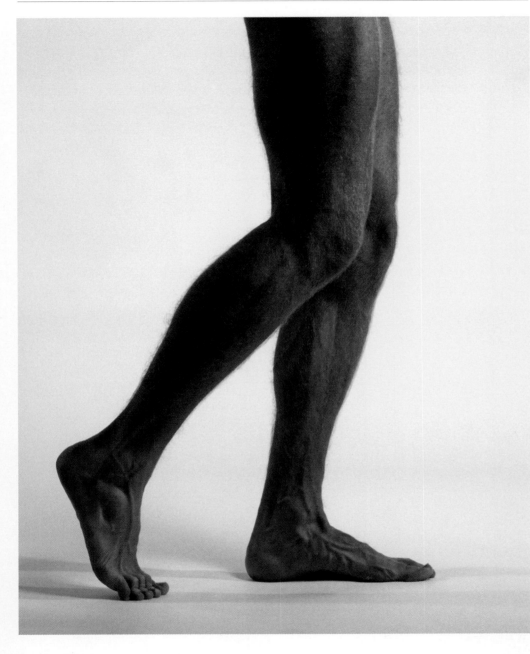

VERTICAL REFLEX THERAPY (VRT}

This is a technique which has proved to be highly successful with back, hip and knee problems. You will be asked to stand while treatment is given. This weight-bearing position permits deeper access to reflexes, which can be painful, but the whole session lasts only 15 minutes. Used in conjunction with osteopathy, results can be dramatic and lasting.

Far right: zonal aromatic therapy involves work on the head and face. One reflexologist gives her clients a facial first so, if you feel like being pampered, this could be for you.

Below: synergistic reflexology involves the simultaneous working of reflexes on the hands and feet.

SYNERGISTIC REFLEXOLOGY (SR)

Another new method involves the simultaneous working of reflexes on the hands and feet. In some cases this produces remarkable results. What's more, it's possible that you may be able to learn to use this therapy on yourself. If you don't fancy the pain of vertical reflex therapy or if it doesn't get results for you, synergistic reflexology is worth trying.

ZONAL AROMATIC THERAPY

Strictly speaking, this may not be classed as a form of reflexology. The system involves work on the head and face. Since this area is one of the body's extremities, it offers another site for accessing energy zones. Acupressure is also included in this therapy to treat migraine and offer relief from stress. One reflexologist gives her clients a facial first so, if you feel like being pampered, this could be for you.

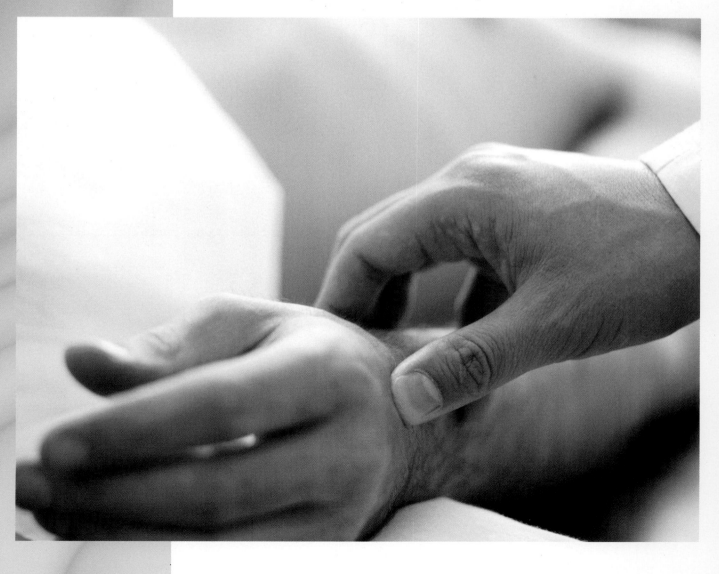

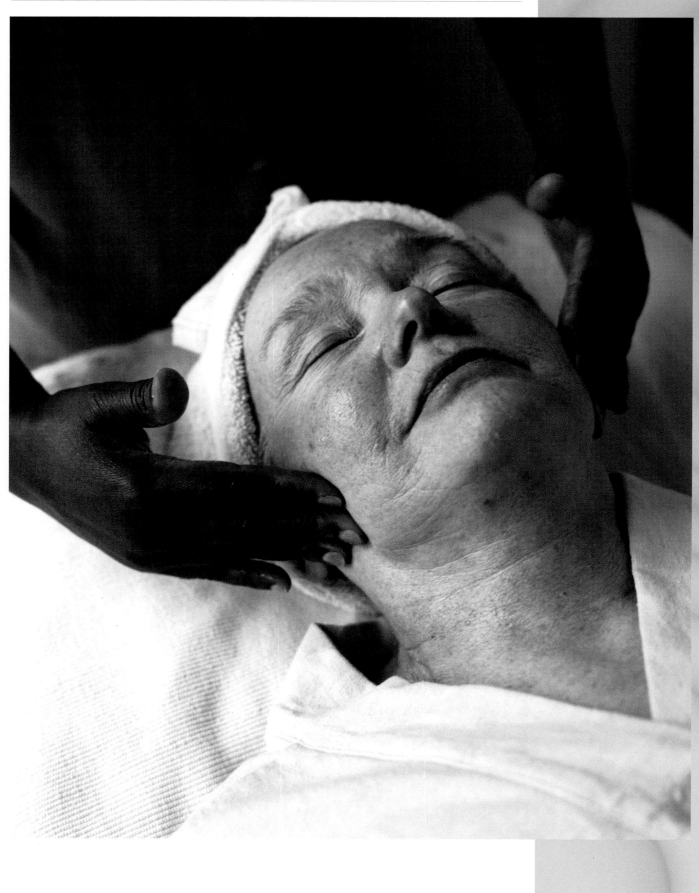

Right: metamorphic technique can release physical and emotional blocks established during the first nine months of life in the womb.

METAMORPHIC TECHNIQUE

This approach uses gentle massage of the feet, hands and head with the aim of releasing physical and emotional blocks established during the first nine months of life in the womb. It was introduced in the 1960s by a British reflexologist, Robert St John. Like reflexology, it is based on the belief that the body is reflected in the feet and hands.

The technique encourages a positive approach to life and has been known to effect a complete "transformation" for people who cannot shake off long standing-problems.

Below: metamorphic technique uses gentle massage of the feet, hands and head.

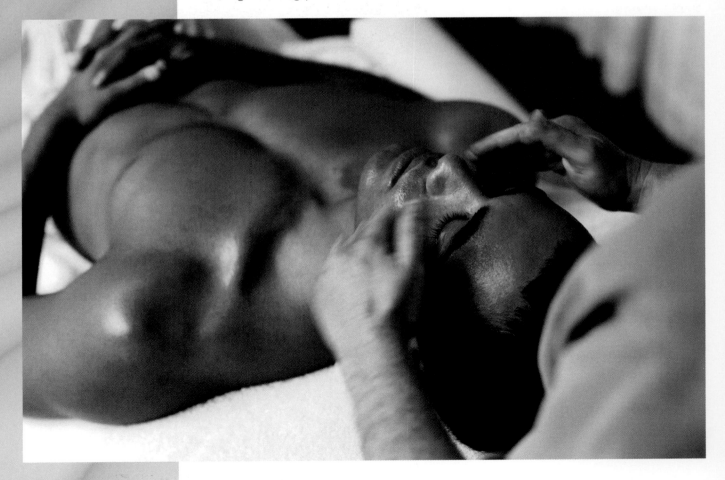

COMPLEMENTARY THERAPIES

Reflexology can be combined with several other complementary therapies to achieve good results. Your practitioner may employ **colour therapy**, asking you to visualise certain colours during the massage. When he is working on your heels, think of red to enhance your personal development. For the balls of the feet, green will harmonise all aspects of your life. Purple, visualised when he works on your toes, helps produce peace of mind and clear thinking.

Crystal healing is another useful addition to the treatment. It can be as simple as holding a piece of rose quartz in each hand during reflexology. Since this particular crystal symbolises love, you may well find this a soothing experience.

Left: your practitioner may employ colour therapy.

Below: crystal healing is another useful addition to the treatment.

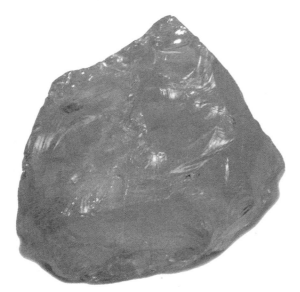

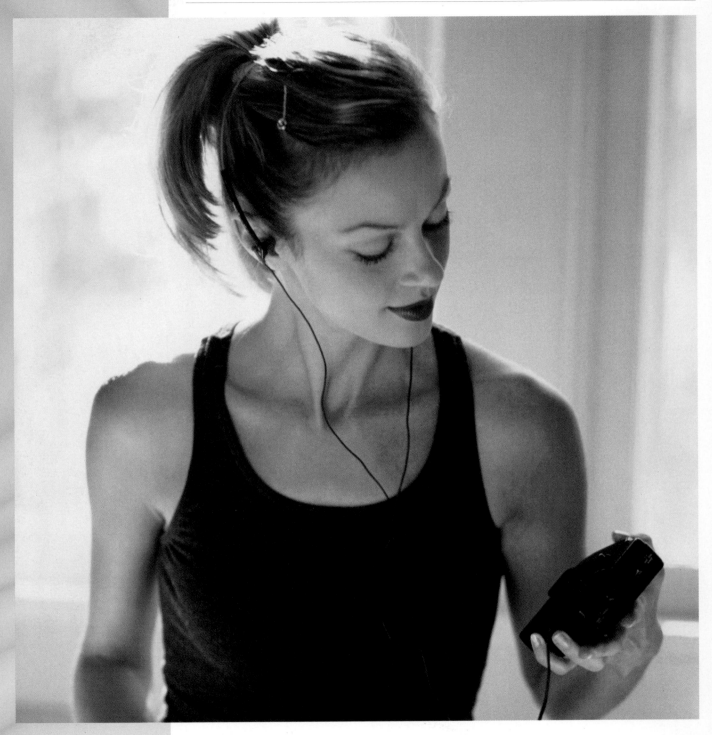

Above: music is often used to bring about relaxation for your body, mind and spirit.

Music is often used to bring about relaxation for your body, mind and spirit. It would be impossible to suggest any particular type from the huge variety available. Your therapist will probably have his own favourites, but will be happy if you choose to take along your own preferences.

Aromatherapy oils can have a therapeutic effect. Your practitioner is unlikely to use them on your feet during treatment, but fragrant oils are often burned in the consulting room to perfume the air and produce a restful ambience.

Below: fragrant oils are often burned in the consulting room to perfume the air.

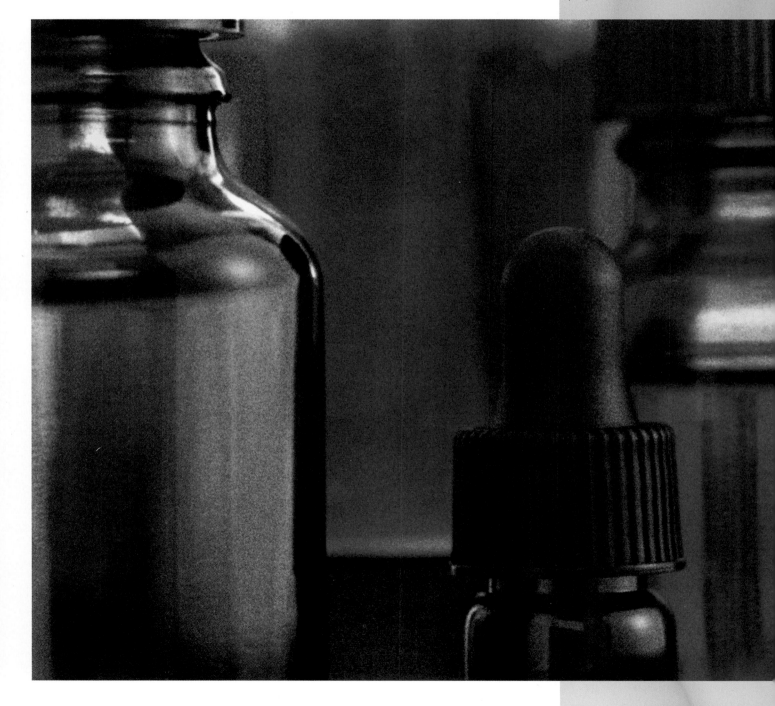

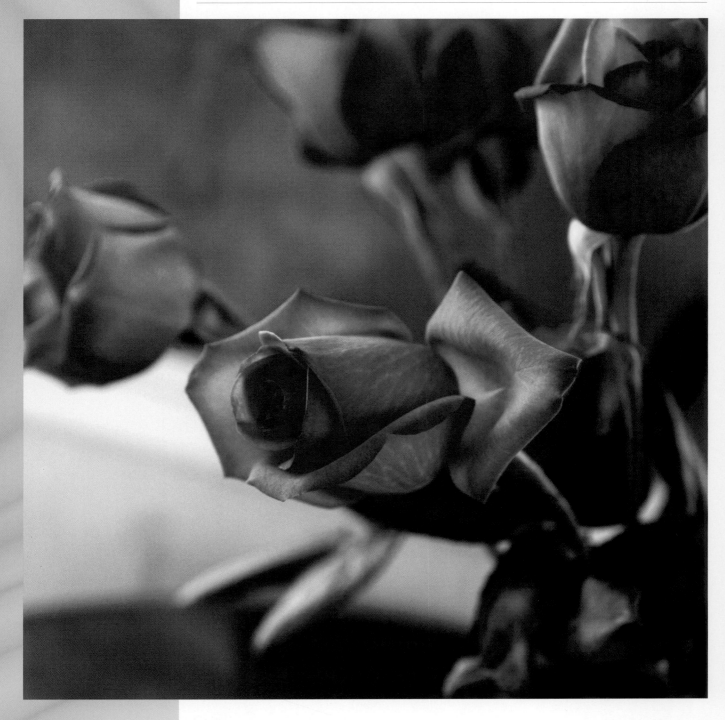

Right: flower remedies are renowned for providing relaxation and relief from stress.

Flower remedies are renowned for providing relaxation and relief from stress, whatever the cause may be. Several companies produce these, but the Bach remedies are probably the most well-known. In particular, Rescue Remedy can be invaluable for coping with any anxiety you may feel about your first consultation with a reflexologist.

Several other complementary therapies combine well with reflexology, but do consult your practitioner about which one to use. It's possible to have too much of a good thing and one type of treatment could hinder or even cancel out another.

Undoubtedly, most complementary therapies are safe. Even so, it's advisable to check with the relevant professional organisation or practitioners' association to make sure. If this is not possible, then have the treatment at an established and reputable health centre. In fact, some complementary therapies are now obtainable through the National Health Service. Ask your doctor what is available in your area.

Remember, too, that you play a decisive part in any treatment you receive. You must be ready to accept healing. This may seem obvious. The fact remains that there are some people who drift from one therapy to another, always in search of the one that will transform their lives (preferably overnight).

Accept that you're a fallible human being. None of us can hope to achieve perfection in any aspect of our lives, but you can – and should – adopt a positive attitude that will enable you to gain the best possible results from any therapy you undertake.

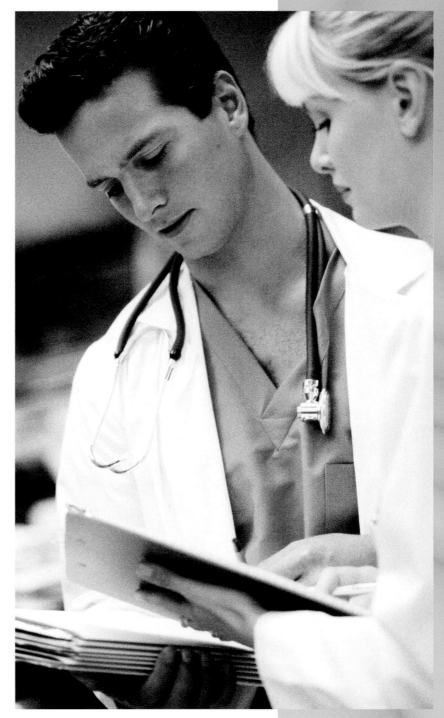

Below: some complementary therapies are now obtainable through the National Health Service.

YOUR QUESTIONS ANSWERED

Q) Is reflexology a medically approved treatment?

A) There is no clinical proof of the claims made for reflexology, but most doctors agree that the treatment is beneficial.

Q) Are there any conditions in which reflexology should not be used?

A) Yes, a few. You should not have reflexology treatment:
if you have thyroid problems
if you have diabetes
if you suffer from epilepsy
if you have thrombosis or phlebitis
if you are in the early stages of pregnancy
if you have arthritis in the feet
if you have osteoporosis
if you have heart problems
if you are taking medication
if you are under the care of a doctor
Should any of these situations apply, you must consult your doctor before undertaking reflexology treatment. If he agrees that you should go ahead, do remember to tell your therapist about the condition from which you are suffering.

Below: if you are pregnant,, you must consult your doctor before undertaking reflexology treatment.

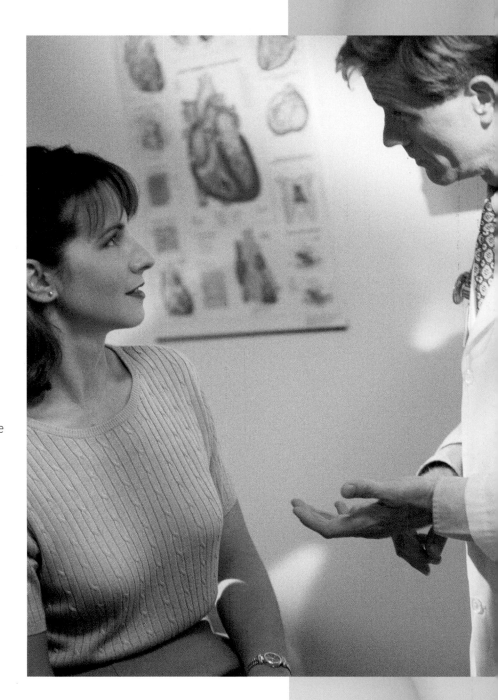

Below: if you exhibit severe symptoms of any kind, you should certainly tell your doctor.

Q) Should I always see my doctor before having reflexology?

A) If you are using reflexology as an aid to relaxation or as preventive treatment, there is no need to consult your doctor beforehand. However, if you exhibit severe symptoms of any kind, you should certainly tell him. In any case, though, your reflexologist will advise you to seek medical help if he considers this to be desirable.

Q) Can I combine reflexology with other complementary therapies?

A) Usually such a combination is perfectly safe. Even so, you should inform all therapists who are giving you treatment. There is a slight possibility that one type of treatment could cancel out another.

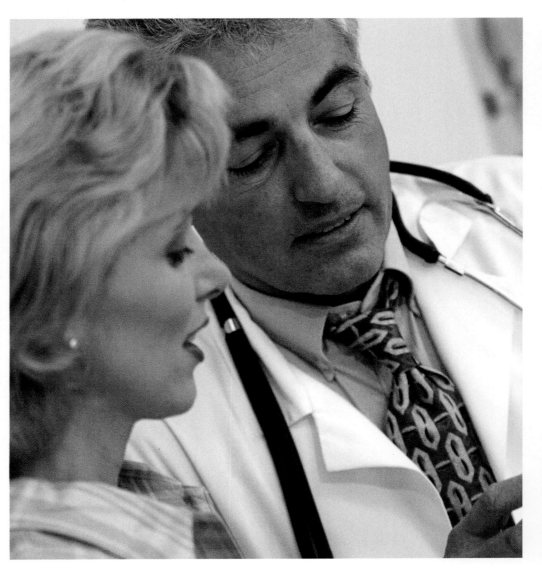

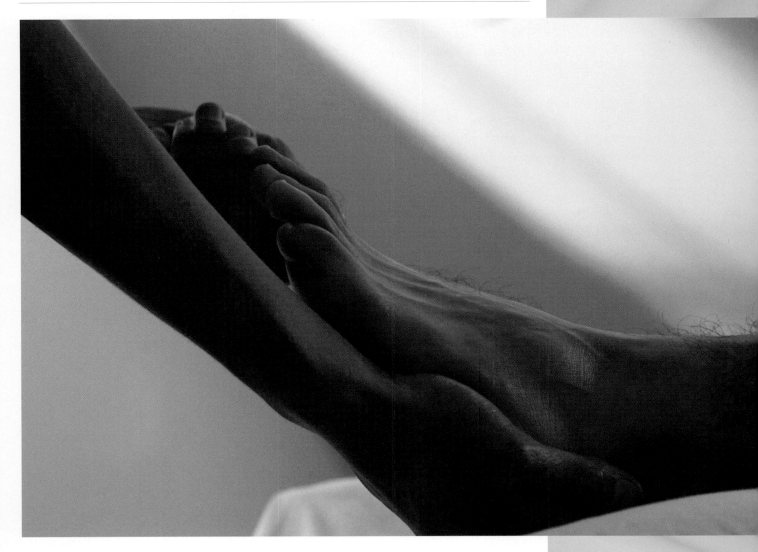

Q) I have heard that reflexology can be painful. Is this true?

A) In general, reflexology is relaxing rather than painful. If you do feel pain when your reflexologist touches a certain area in the foot, this probably indicates a blockage. He will need to work this area in order to clear the blockage, but you are most unlikely to feel more than a little discomfort – and even this will be short-lived.

Q) How many sessions will I need?

A) This depends on several factors and you should rely on your therapist to advise you. It is desirable to have at least three treatments, even if your problems seem to have cleared up after the first session. Conversely, if no improvement is apparent, your reflexologist may then suggest that you try some other form of complementary treatment.

Above: if you feel pain when your reflexologist touches a certain area in the foot, this probably indicates a blockage.

Far right and below: in serious conditions such as those mentioned above, pain control can be one of the most beneficial outcomes of reflexology treatments.

Q) If my problem appears to be cured by reflexology, is it likely to recur at some future date?

A) This can happen with certain conditions. Your practitioner will be able to advise you about ways to prevent this.

It is important to remember that no reputable reflexologist will ever claim to cure any condition. "Cures" are invariably claimed by the patient, not the practitioner.

Q) Can reflexology be used as a preventive therapy?

A) Definitely. Having once experienced the benefits of a course of reflexology treatment, many patients return for a "top-up" at regular intervals. This ensures that the correct energy flow is maintained throughout the body. It also ensures that minor problems can be dealt with before they develop into major ones.

Q) Can reflexology help in cases of terminal illness?

A) Yes. Obviously the treatment cannot cure such illnesses or remove their cause, but it does improve the patient's quality of life. In addition to the relaxation so often mentioned in this book, reflexology can significantly improve the patient's outlook by producing a marked improvement in the general condition. In turn, this usually helps towards better digestive function and sounder sleep.

Q) What about pain control? Can reflexology help with this?

A) Yes. In serious conditions such as those mentioned above, pain control can be one of the most beneficial outcomes of reflexology treatments. Briefly – the body produces its own pain-killers, known as endorphins. During the treatment, the therapist applies pressure to certain reflex areas. These can stimulate the brain into releasing more endorphins. Since these are known to be at least five times more powerful than morphine, the pain relief can be noticeable.

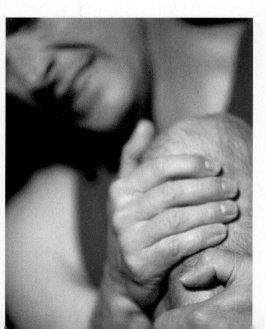

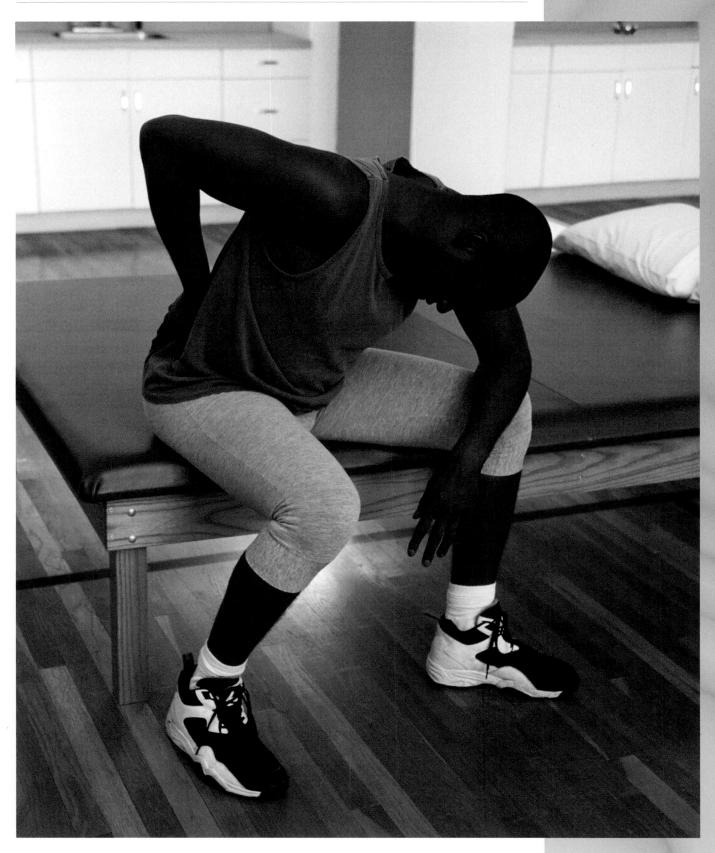

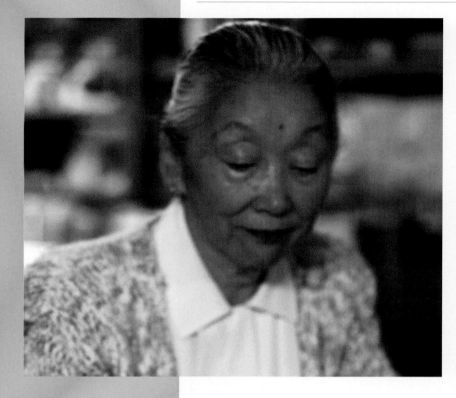

Above and below: senior citizens and babies can gain tremendous benefit from reflexology.

Q) Can elderly people benefit from reflexology treatment?

A) Yes. Senior citizens can gain tremendous benefit from reflexology. See page 32 for details of the tests carried out in Manchester.

Q) What about babies and children?

A) Obviously, the treatment given to children differs slightly from that offered to adults, but it is absolutely safe for them to be treated by a qualified reflexologist. Such treatment must be given by a professional practitioner and you should not attempt it yourself. It is worth knowing, though, that it is perfectly safe – and very effective – to gently stroke the feet of a fractious baby.

Q) Is reflexology especially effective with any particular ailment?

A) Reflexology is usually successful in treating any condition which needs to be balanced or regulated. For instance, it works well with menstrual irregularity, irritable bowel syndrome and digestive problems. It's generally useful, too, in dealing with everyday common ailments like headaches, catarrh, and cramp.

In fact, though reflexology is not in any way a "cure all", it has been found to be helpful in at least some aspect of practically all conditions.

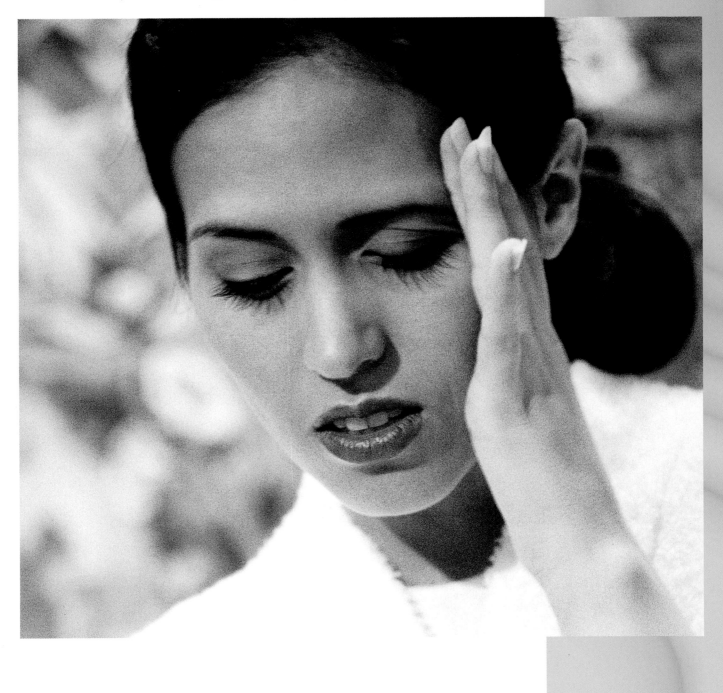

Below: it's generally useful in dealing with everyday common ailments like headaches.

Q) Does this include nervous disorders?

A) Very much so. As stated at the beginning of this book, 70% of hospital beds are occupied by patients with stress-related problems. In other words, tensions in the mind are reflected in the state of the body. Reflexology helps by releasing these tensions and, in consequence, relaxing and relieving physical problems.

Q) I don't fully understand the term "holistic approach". Can you explain?

A) The word "holistic" is derived from the Greek term "holos", which means whole. Thus, the holistic approach is one which seeks to deal with the whole person – body, mind and spirit – rather than with just one part of the body. It is safe to say that if there is dis-ease in one part of the body other parts will almost certainly be affected. Similarly, as we have already seen, dis-ease in the mind (in the shape of stress, anxiety etc.) can produce physical problems. And most people would surely agree that mental and physical difficulties produce an element of spiritual discomfort. Thus the term holistic approach simply indicates that treatment is given to the whole person, aiming to produce a perfect balance between the three aspects of the self.

Below: seventy per cent of hospital beds are occupied by patients with stress-related problems.

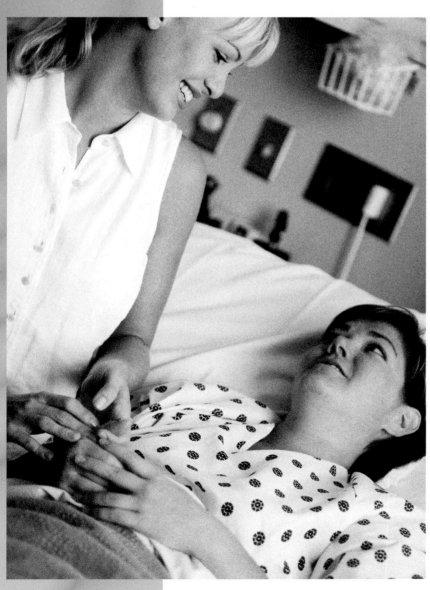

APPENDIX

Useful Addresses

The Association of Reflexologists
27 Old Gloucester Street
London WC1N 3XX

The British School of Reflexology
Holistic Healing Centre
92 Sheering Road
Old Harlow
Essex CM17 0JW

The British Reflexology Association
Monks Orchard
Whitbourne
Worcester WR6 5RB

Further Reading

Reflexology: a step-by-step guide
Ann Gillanders, Gaia Books Ltd, 1995.

Healing with Reflexology
Rosalind Oxenford, Gill and Macmillan,
1996.

Reflexology
Chris Stormer, Teach Yourself Books,
1996.

*The Complete Illustrated Guide to
Reflexology*
Inge Dougans, Element Books, 1996.

Principles of Reflexology
Nicola Hall, Thorsons, 1996.

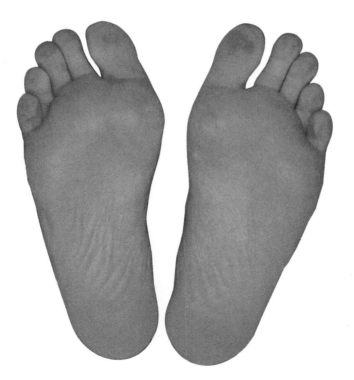

INDEX

INDEX

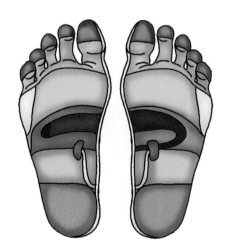

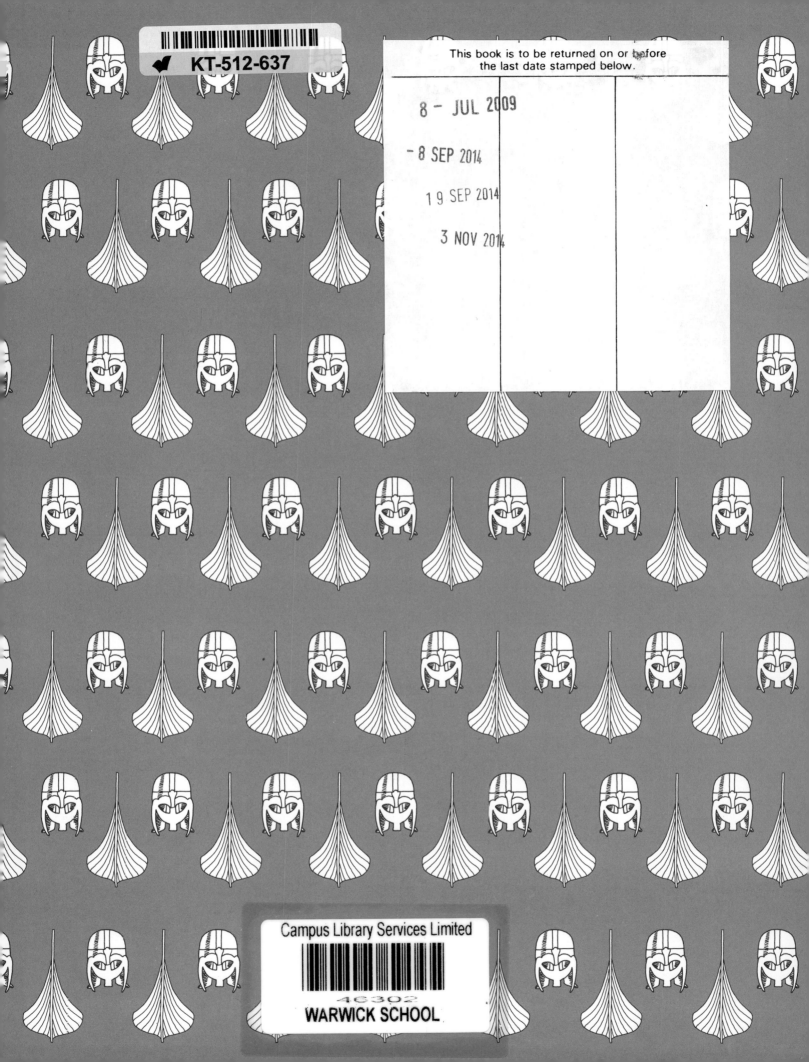

DORLING KINDERSLEY 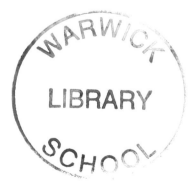 EYEWITNESS GUIDES

VIKING

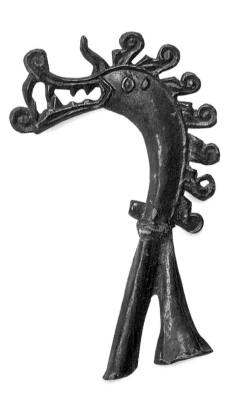

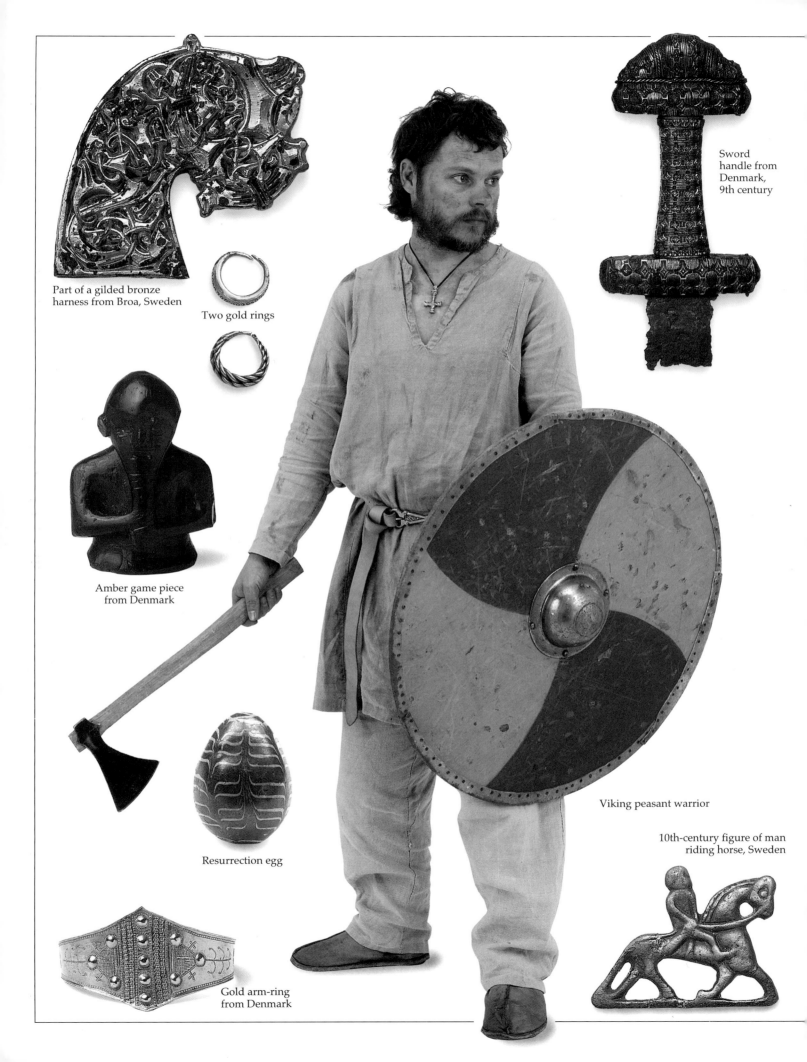

Part of a gilded bronze harness from Broa, Sweden

Two gold rings

Amber game piece from Denmark

Resurrection egg

Gold arm-ring from Denmark

Sword handle from Denmark, 9th century

Viking peasant warrior

10th-century figure of man riding horse, Sweden

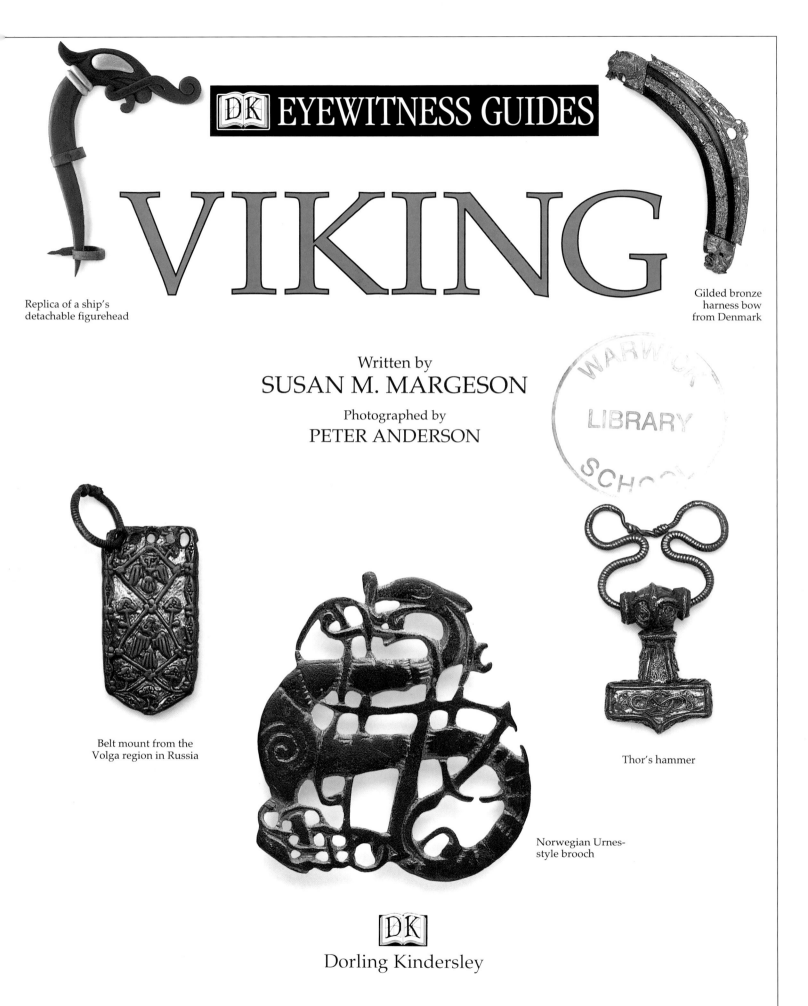

DK EYEWITNESS GUIDES

VIKING

Replica of a ship's
detachable figurehead

Gilded bronze
harness bow
from Denmark

Written by
SUSAN M. MARGESON

Photographed by
PETER ANDERSON

Belt mount from the
Volga region in Russia

Thor's hammer

Norwegian Urnes-
style brooch

DK
Dorling Kindersley

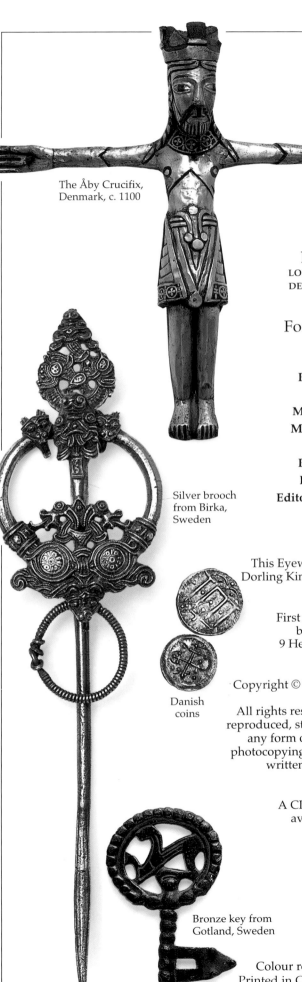

The Åby Crucifix,
Denmark, c. 1100

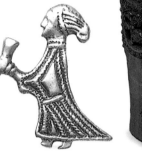

Animal-head post from
the Oseberg ship-burial,
Norway, c. 800–850

Dorling Kindersley

LONDON, NEW YORK, AUCKLAND,
DELHI, JOHANNESBURG, MUNICH,
PARIS and SYDNEY

For a full catalogue, visit
DK www.dk.com

Silver pendant of a
Viking woman

Silver brooch
from Birka,
Sweden

Project editor Scott Steedman
Art editor Andrew Nash
Managing editor Simon Adams
Managing art editor Julia Harris
Researcher Céline Carez
Production Catherine Semark
Picture research Julia Ruxton
Editorial consultant David M. Wilson

This Eyewitness ® Guide has been conceived by
Dorling Kindersley Limited and Editions Gallimard

First published in Great Britain in 1994
by Dorling Kindersley Limited,
9 Henrietta Street, London WC2E 8PS

6 8 10 9 7 5

Copyright © 1994 Dorling Kindersley Limited, London

Danish
coins

A CIP catalogue record for this book is
available from the British Library.

ISBN 0 7513 6022 8

Colour reproduction by Colourscan, Singapore
Printed in China by Toppan Printing Co., (Shenzhen) Ltd.

Gilded bronze mount from
horse's bridle, Broa, Sweden

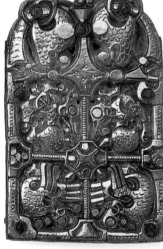

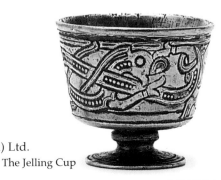

The Jelling Cup

Bronze key from
Gotland, Sweden

Contents

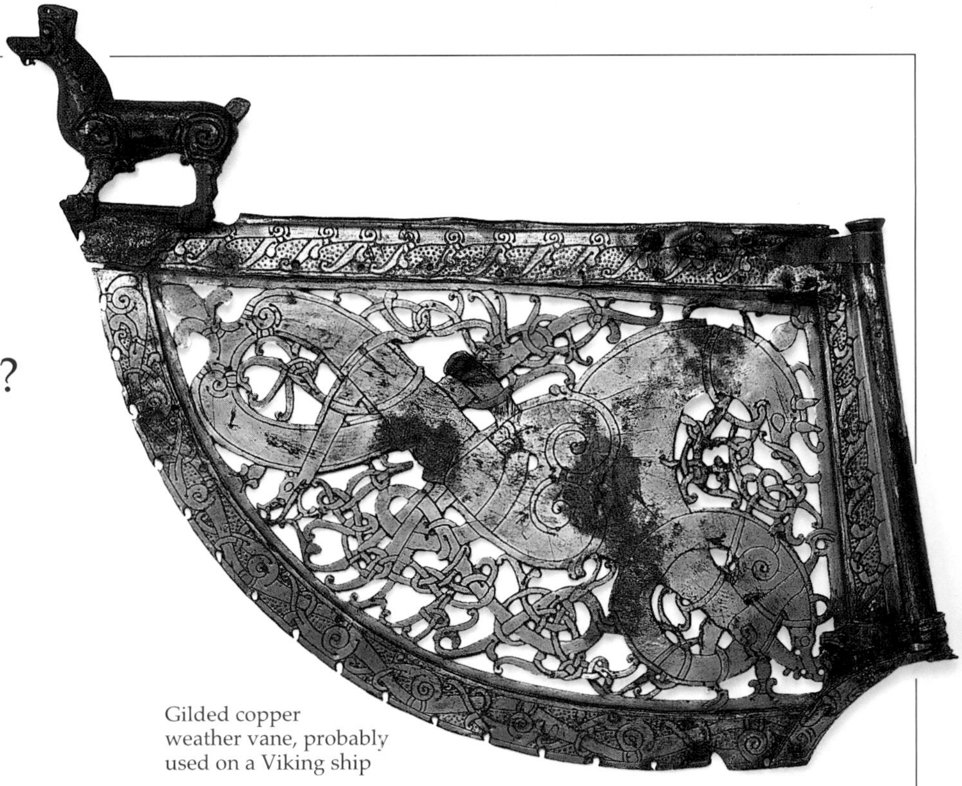

Gilded copper
weather vane, probably
used on a Viking ship

Who were the Vikings?

FOR 300 YEARS, from the 8th to 11th centuries, the Vikings took the world by storm. In search of land, slaves, gold, and silver, these brave warriors and explorers set sail from their homes in Norway, Sweden, and Denmark. They raided all across Europe, voyaged as far as Baghdad, and even reached America. The speed and daring of Viking attacks became legendary. Christian monks wrote with horror about the violent raids on rich monasteries and towns. But the Vikings were more than wild barbarians from the north. They were shrewd traders, excellent navigators, and superb craftsmen and shipbuilders. They had a rich tradition of story-telling, and lived in a society that was open and democratic for its day.

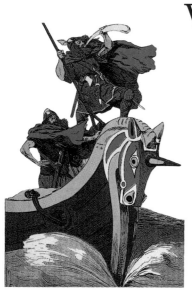

ROMANTIC VIKINGS
There are many romantic fantasies about Vikings. Most of them are wrong! Many pictures show them wearing horned helmets. But real Vikings wore round or pointed caps of iron or leather (p. 13).

CATTY BROOCH
A Swedish Viking held his cloak in place with this brooch. It is made of silver coated in gold. The details are highlighted with niello, a black metallic compound. The style of decoration, with little cat-like heads, is known as the Borre style.

SCARY SHIP
Vikings often carved terrifying beasts on their ships to scare their enemies (p. 10). This dragon head was found in a river bed in Holland. It dates from the 5th century, 300 years before the Viking Age. It may have been part of a Saxon warship sunk during a raid. Sailing ships were known before the Vikings, but they were less sophisticated. Viking ships were fast and flexible, and could cruise up narrow channels and inlets with ease.

THE VIKING WORLD
The brown areas on this map are Viking settlements. From late in the 8th century, Vikings raided, traded, and explored far and wide. They discovered Iceland in 870, and sailed further west to Greenland in 985 (pp. 20–21). Leif the Lucky was probably the first European to set foot on America. He is thought to have landed in Newfoundland, Canada in 1001. In the east, Vikings sailed the Baltic Sea and continued up rivers into Russia. They went on overland as far as Constantinople (now Istanbul) and Jerusalem. Other Vikings sailed around the west coast of Europe and into the Mediterranean Sea. Thanks to their ships and skill at seafaring, they could take people completely by surprise.

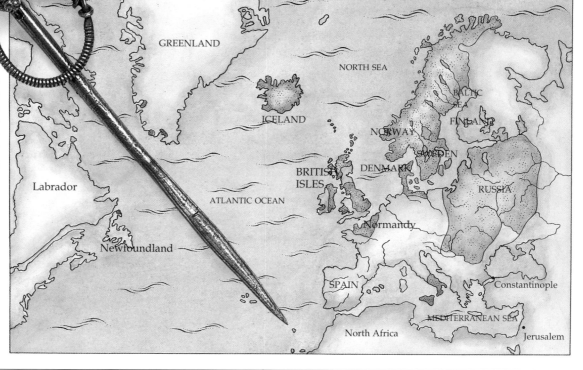

GREENLAND

NORTH SEA

ICELAND

NORWAY

BALTIC SEA

FINLAND

SWEDEN

DENMARK

BRITISH ISLES

Labrador

RUSSIA

ATLANTIC OCEAN

Normandy

Newfoundland

SPAIN

Constantinople

MEDITERRANEAN SEA

North Africa

Jerusalem

**AXE OF
A CHIEFTAIN**

Silver wires in the form of plant shoots

This great iron axehead was found in Mammen, Denmark. It is decorated with silver wires. This side features a glaring human face and a fantastic bird that twists around its own wings, which turn into plant shoots. The Mammen Axe is too beautiful to have been used in battle, and must have been carried by a chieftain to show his power.

Loop so hammer could be worn on chain around neck

THOR'S HAMMER
Vikings believed in many different gods (pp. 52–53). This silver hammer is the sign of the great god Thor. He was said to ride his chariot across the sky, smashing giant snakes with his hammer and making thunder and lightning.

Silver loop for chain

Figure of great bird

GLITTERING SWORD
A strong sword was a Viking's most prized weapon (pp. 14–15). This sword was made and decorated in Norway. Its owner must have died in battle in Ireland, because it was found in a man's grave in Dublin (pp. 54–57). It is beautifully crafted. The hilt and guard are made of copper decorated with layers of gold and twisted silver and copper wires.

Pommel

Grip, once covered in leather

Guard to protect hand

Helmet with bird's crest and beak

Moustache

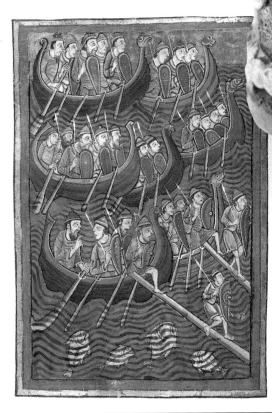

**HERE COME
THE VIKINGS!**
Ivar the Boneless and his army invaded England in 869. This manuscript (made 300 years later) shows ships full of armed warriors arriving at the coast. The first raiders are walking down gangplanks onto the shore. Ivar and his men terrorized the country and killed King Edmund (p. 17).

Mouth

**MYSTERIOUS
VIKING FACE**
Who is this mysterious Viking? A god? A hero from a legend? A warrior? Real pictures of Vikings are very rare. The Vikings didn't have books, and most of the people and animals (pp. 36–37) in their art are imaginary or hard to identify. This small silver head from Aska, Sweden was worn on a chain as a pendant. It may have been meant to warn off enemies or bring good luck.

Iron blade, now rusted

Lords of the sea

THE VIKINGS WERE SUPERB sailors. Their wooden longships carried them across wild seas, riding the waves, dodging rocks and icebergs and surviving storms. In open seas, the Vikings relied on a big, rectangular sail. To manoeuvre in coastal waters and rivers, they dropped the mast and rowed the ship instead. Whenever possible, they sailed within sight of land. Far from the coast, Vikings navigated by the sun and stars. Their knowledge of seabirds, fish, winds, and wave patterns helped them find their way. Wood rots quickly, so there is little left of most longships. But fortunately a few have survived, thanks to the Viking custom of burying rich people in ships (pp. 54–57). The best preserved are the Oseberg and Gokstad ships from Norway. Both are slender, elegant vessels, light but surprisingly strong.

Stem-post or prow

Ship is made of light oak wood with heavier mast of pine

Sixteen strakes (planks) on each side, each one over-lapping the strake below

Sixteen oarports (holes) on each side

GOKSTAD SHIP, FRONT VIEW
One of the grandest Viking ships was found at Gokstad, beside Oslo Fjord in Norway. It was excavated in 1880. The elegant lines of the prow and strakes (planks) show the skill of the ship-builders. The ship is 23.2 m (76 ft) long and 5.2 m (17 ft) wide. The keel is a single piece of oak, cut from a tree at least 25 m (82 ft) tall!

Keel

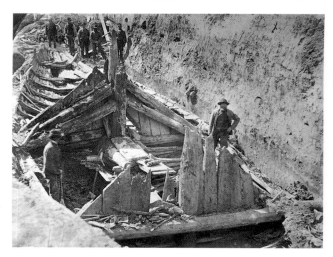

DIGGING OUT THE SHIP
The Norwegian ships were preserved by unusual wet conditions. The Gokstad ship sat in a large mound with a burial chamber on its deck. The skeleton of a man lay in the chamber, surrounded by his worldly possessions. He had been buried around 900 A.D.

SAILING TO THE WINDY CITY
The Gokstad ship had 32 shields on each side, painted yellow and black alternately. A full-size replica was sailed across the Atlantic Ocean to Chicago in 1893. It proved how seaworthy the real ship must have been.

Gunwale (top strake)

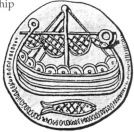

LEARNING THE ROPES
Coins and picture stones give clues about how Viking ships were rigged (roped) and sailed. This coin from Birka, Sweden shows a ship with a furled (rolled-up) sail.

Mast

Mast fish, to lock mast in place

Deck boards

RAISING THE GOKSTAD MAST
The heavy mast was lowered into a groove in the keelson and held in place by the mast fish. The deck boards were loose, so the sailors could store their belongings under them.

Strakes

Keelson, which runs above keel

Keel

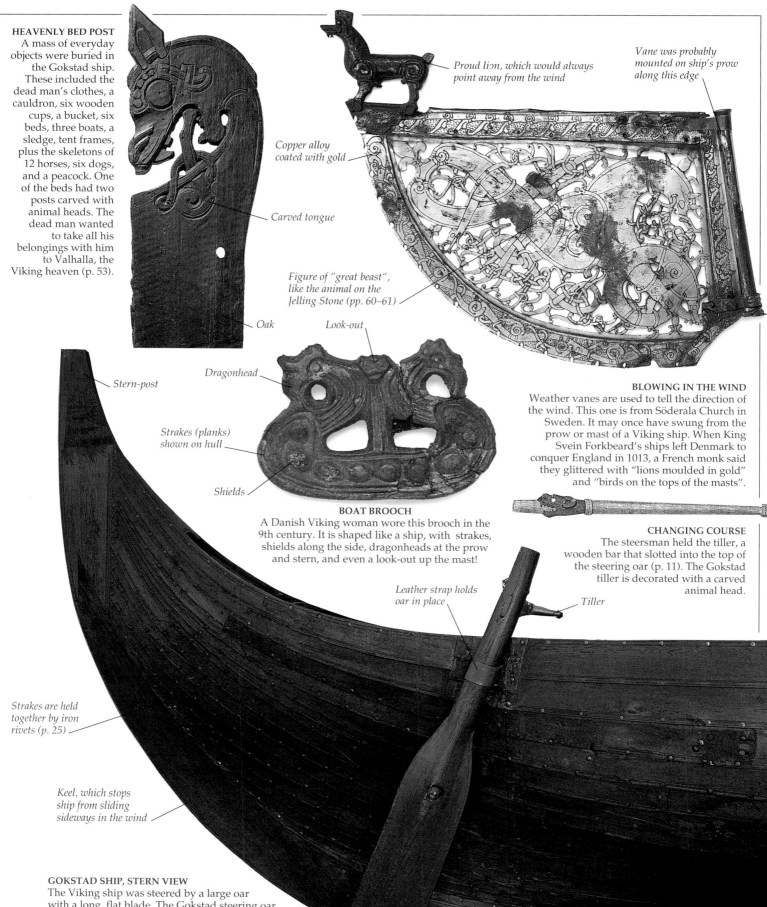

HEAVENLY BED POST
A mass of everyday objects were buried in the Gokstad ship. These included the dead man's clothes, a cauldron, six wooden cups, a bucket, six beds, three boats, a sledge, tent frames, plus the skeletons of 12 horses, six dogs, and a peacock. One of the beds had two posts carved with animal heads. The dead man wanted to take all his belongings with him to Valhalla, the Viking heaven (p. 53).

Carved tongue

Oak

Proud lion, which would always point away from the wind

Copper alloy coated with gold

Figure of "great beast", like the animal on the Jelling Stone (pp. 60–61)

Vane was probably mounted on ship's prow along this edge

BLOWING IN THE WIND
Weather vanes are used to tell the direction of the wind. This one is from Söderala Church in Sweden. It may once have swung from the prow or mast of a Viking ship. When King Svein Forkbeard's ships left Denmark to conquer England in 1013, a French monk said they glittered with "lions moulded in gold" and "birds on the tops of the masts".

Stern-post

Dragonhead

Look-out

Strakes (planks) shown on hull

Shields

BOAT BROOCH
A Danish Viking woman wore this brooch in the 9th century. It is shaped like a ship, with strakes, shields along the side, dragonheads at the prow and stern, and even a look-out up the mast!

CHANGING COURSE
The steersman held the tiller, a wooden bar that slotted into the top of the steering oar (p. 11). The Gokstad tiller is decorated with a carved animal head.

Leather strap holds oar in place

Tiller

Strakes are held together by iron rivets (p. 25)

Keel, which stops ship from sliding sideways in the wind

GOKSTAD SHIP, STERN VIEW
The Viking ship was steered by a large oar with a long, flat blade. The Gokstad steering oar is 3.3 m (10 ft 9 in) long. The steering oar was always attached to the right side of the ship near the stern. In English, a ship's right side is still called starboard, after the old Norse word *styra* (to steer). The Gokstad ship is symmetrical – the prow is identical to the stern, except that it has no steering oar.

Steering oar

A Viking warship

LIGHT AND SLENDER, the Viking warship carried warriors far across the ocean. It was the longest, slenderest, and quickest Viking vessel. Like other longships, the warship had a sail and mast, but could also be rowed. Depending on its size, it needed from 24 to 50 oars. On long voyages, the Viking warriors rowed in shifts. They could glide their ship up narrow inlets and land on any flat beach. Even when it was full, the warship had such a shallow keel that it did not need a jetty or quay, and could be unloaded right on the shore. Some of the ships on the Bayeux Tapestry (below) carry horses as well as warriors. When beached, both animals and men could wade ashore. Two well-preserved warships were discovered in the Roskilde Fjord in Denmark. They had been filled with stones and deliberately sunk around the year 1000. The longest one is 28 m (92 ft) from prow to stern, making it the longest Viking ship ever found.

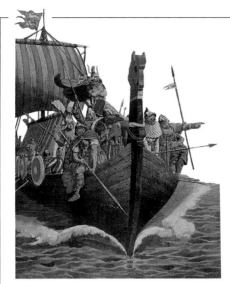

UNWELCOME GUESTS
A ship full of fierce warriors suddenly landing on the beach filled people with fear and horror. This highly romanticized picture of raiders appeared in a French magazine in 1911.

Dragon made of carved and painted pine wood

Detachable wooden figurehead

DANISH DRAGON SHIP
In 1962, five Viking ships were excavated from Roskilde Fjord in Sjælland, Denmark. They had been scuttled (sunk deliberately), probably to block a channel and protect the harbour from enemy ships. This is a reconstruction of one of the warships. It was 17.4 m (57 ft) long and only 2.6 m (8 ft 6 in) across at the widest point. The ship had seven strakes (planks) on each side, the top three made of ash, the bottom four of oak. There were 12 oarports (holes) on each side, so 24 men could row together.

Leather thong holds figurehead in place

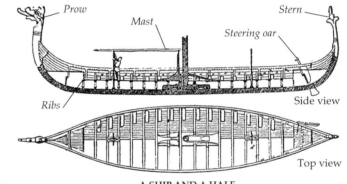

Prow *Mast* *Stern* *Steering oar*

Ribs *Side view*

Top view

A SHIP AND A HALF
Cross beams and ribs helped to strengthen the hull of a Viking ship. The gaps between the strakes were stuffed with tarred wool. This is called caulking. It kept the water out, and made the ship more flexible in rough seas.

Original rope may have been made of walrus skin *Mooring post*

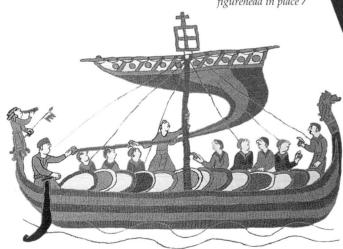

WILLIAM'S WARSHIP
The Normans were descended from Vikings who settled in Normandy in France (p. 16). The Bayeux Tapestry describes their conquest of England in 1066. In this scene, the proud ship of the Norman leader William the Conqueror sails towards England. A look-out in the stern blows a horn, while the steersman holds the tiller, attached to the steering oar. The ship has an animal head prow, and shields line its sides.

Hull made of seven slender strakes (planks)

Each strake overlaps the one below, in a technique called "clinker" boat-building

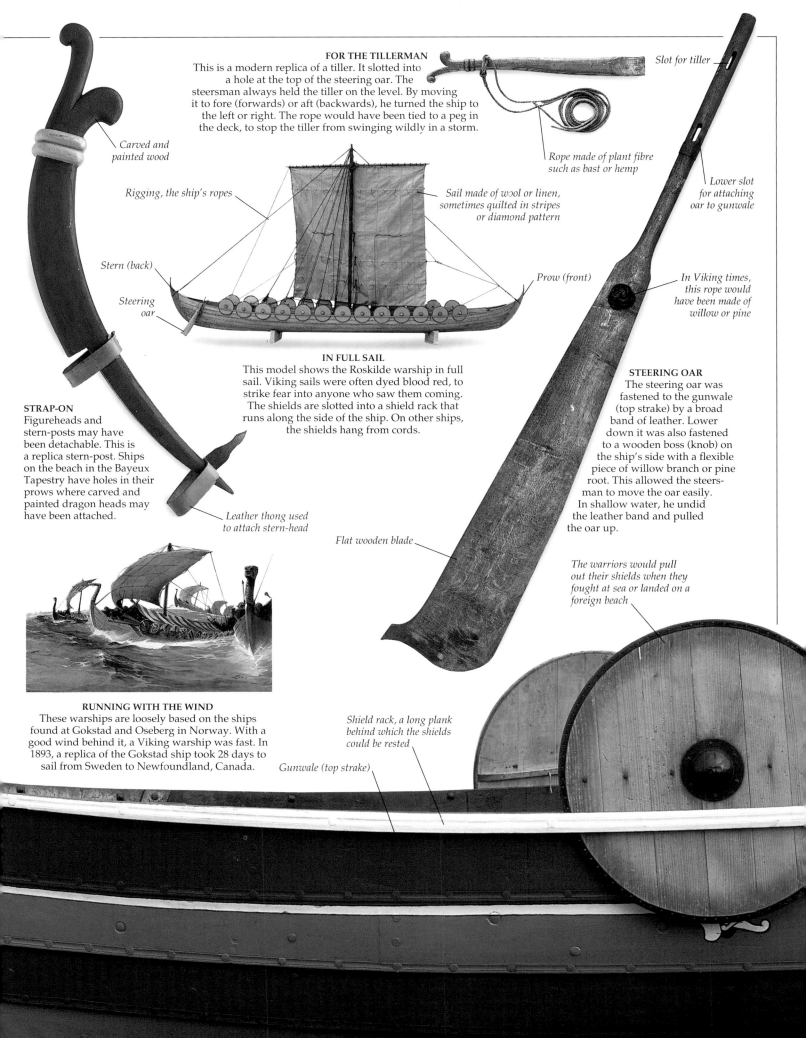

FOR THE TILLERMAN
This is a modern replica of a tiller. It slotted into a hole at the top of the steering oar. The steersman always held the tiller on the level. By moving it to fore (forwards) or aft (backwards), he turned the ship to the left or right. The rope would have been tied to a peg in the deck, to stop the tiller from swinging wildly in a storm.

Slot for tiller

Rope made of plant fibre such as bast or hemp

Lower slot for attaching oar to gunwale

Carved and painted wood

Rigging, the ship's ropes

Sail made of wool or linen, sometimes quilted in stripes or diamond pattern

Stern (back)

Steering oar

Prow (front)

In Viking times, this rope would have been made of willow or pine

IN FULL SAIL
This model shows the Roskilde warship in full sail. Viking sails were often dyed blood red, to strike fear into anyone who saw them coming. The shields are slotted into a shield rack that runs along the side of the ship. On other ships, the shields hang from cords.

STEERING OAR
The steering oar was fastened to the gunwale (top strake) by a broad band of leather. Lower down it was also fastened to a wooden boss (knob) on the ship's side with a flexible piece of willow branch or pine root. This allowed the steersman to move the oar easily. In shallow water, he undid the leather band and pulled the oar up.

STRAP-ON
Figureheads and stern-posts may have been detachable. This is a replica stern-post. Ships on the beach in the Bayeux Tapestry have holes in their prows where carved and painted dragon heads may have been attached.

Leather thong used to attach stern-head

Flat wooden blade

The warriors would pull out their shields when they fought at sea or landed on a foreign beach

RUNNING WITH THE WIND
These warships are loosely based on the ships found at Gokstad and Oseberg in Norway. With a good wind behind it, a Viking warship was fast. In 1893, a replica of the Gokstad ship took 28 days to sail from Sweden to Newfoundland, Canada.

Shield rack, a long plank behind which the shields could be rested

Gunwale (top strake)

Viking warriors

THE TRUE SPIRIT OF THE VIKING AGE was daring courage. To the Viking warrior, honour and glory in battle were the only things that lasted forever. A warrior had to be ready to follow his lord or king into battle or on a raid or expedition. As a member of a loyal band of followers, known as a *lið*, he could be called up to fight at any moment. In the later Viking Age, kings had the power to raise a force (or *leiðang*) of ships, men, supplies, and weapons. The kingdom was divided into small units, and each unit provided one warrior. Groups of units donated a ship to carry the warriors on a raid to far-away lands.

ARCHER IN ACTION
Vikings were skilled with bow and arrow, both in battle and hunting. A well-preserved bow was found in Hedeby, the great Danish Viking town (now in Germany). It was made of yew wood. A rich boat burial in Hedeby contained a bundle of arrows with bronze mounts. They probably belonged to a nobleman.

Bow made of flexible wood such as yew

Fur hat

Shaft of flexible birch wood

Flights, pieces of bird feather added to stabilize arrow in air

Sharp iron arrowhead

Bear-tooth pendant

Bowstring of twisted fibres

Bundle of arrows

Leather quiver, a pouch for holding arrows

Leather sheath for knife

BOUND FOR GLORY
In this romantic engraving, warriors fight with axe and sword. The Viking poem *Hávamál* says:
"Cattle die
kindred die,
every man is mortal:
but I know one thing
that never dies,
The glory of the
great dead."

Round shield

Sword

Conical helmet

Spear

STONE WARRIOR
This Viking warrior was carved in the 10th century on a stone cross in Middleton, Yorkshire, England. His weapons are laid out around him, as they would have been in a traditional burial (pp. 54–57). The Anglo-Saxon poem *The Battle of Maldon* describes the noise and fury of a battle between Danish Vikings and the English: "Then they let the spears, hard as a file, go from their hands; let the darts (arrows), ground sharp, fly; bows were busy; shield received point; bitter was the rush of battle."

Axe

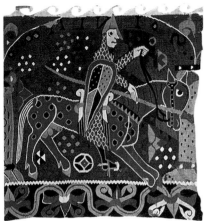

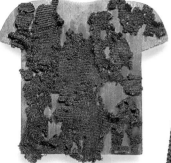

THE LATEST FASHION
Vikings usually fought on foot. Fashions changed in the late 11th century, at the end of the Viking Age, when cavalry began to be used in battle. This mounted warrior comes from a tapestry woven in Baldishol, Norway around the year 1200. He is wearing a helmet and chain-mail tunic, and carrying a kite-shaped shield. These longer shields protected the body better than round ones.

Iron spearhead

Iron plates welded together

Chain mail may have hung from back to protect neck

REAL HELMET (NO HORNS)
The typical Viking helmet was shaped like this one from Gjermundbu in Norway. It has "goggles" to protect the eyes.

Iron helmet with noseguard

Wooden shaft

Chain mail to protect neck

Brooch

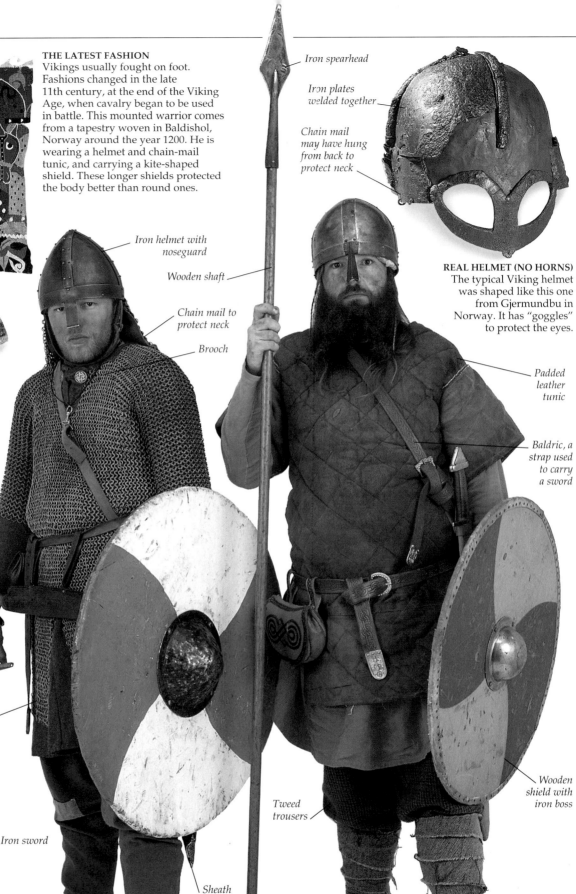

ONE HEAVY SHIRT
These fragments of a chain-mail shirt come from Gjermundbu, Norway. Making chain mail was a slow job. Each iron ring had to be forged separately. Then it was linked to the last one and closed with a rivet or welded in place. It took thousands of rings to make one shirt.

Padded leather tunic

Baldric, a strap used to carry a sword

Sword guard to protect hand

Chain-mail tunic, long enough to cover waist

Iron sword

CASUAL DRESS
Unlike Roman legionaries or modern soldiers, Viking warriors didn't wear uniforms. Every soldier had to dress and arm himself. Iron helmets were worn by chieftains – poor warriors had to make do with leather caps, which didn't offer as much protection. Some wore leather tunics instead of chain mail. Wooden shields were held up against arrows and blows from axes or swords.

Tweed trousers

Sheath for sword

Wooden shield with iron boss

Men probably wore woollen socks, like one found in York, England

Leather shoes, often made of goat skin

Weapons

His spear, his axe, his shield, and especially his sword – these were a warrior's most prized possessions. In poems and sagas (pp. 52–53), swords were given names celebrating the strength and sharpness of the blade or the glittering decoration of the hilt (handle). Weapons were made of iron, often decorated with inlaid or encrusted silver or copper. A beautifully ornamented sword was a sign that the owner was rich or powerful. Before the arrival of Christianity, a Viking's weapons were usually buried with him when he died. Helmets (p. 13) are rarely found, because most of them were made of leather and have rotted away.

Notch to cut feathers

Broad iron blade

Wooden board about 1 m (3 ft) in diameter

Leather binding to protect the edges

ARROWS
Arrows were used for hunting as well as battle (p. 12). These iron arrow-heads from Norway would have been lashed to shafts of birch wood. The two on the right were used to hunt reindeer. The other one was designed for killing birds.

THRUSTING AND THROWING
Spears were mainly used as thrusting weapons, and had large broad blades. The sockets were often decorated. Throwing spears had much lighter, narrower blades, so they would fly straight and true.

Geometric patterns of copper and silver

Wooden shaft was riveted into socket

BERSERK
Tyr was the Viking god of war. In this romantic engraving he has a shaggy bear-skin cloak, with the bear's head worn as a helmet. Warriors called *berserkir* prepared for battle by putting on bearskin cloaks or shirts and working themselves into a frenzy. This was called going *berserk*, from the Old Norse word meaning "bear shirt".

Iron thrusting spearhead from Ronnesbæksholm, Sjælland, Denmark

Iron throwing spearhead from Fyrkat fortress, Jutland, Denmark

SHIELD

Viking shields were round and made of wood. Unfortunately, wood rots quickly, and very few shields have survived. This one is a replica based on fragments found with the Roskilde warship (pp. 10–11). The iron boss in the centre protected the warrior's hand. He held the shield by a grip on the other side of the boss. Shields were often covered in leather or painted in bright colours. A Viking poem, *Ragnarsdrápa*, even describes a shield painted with pictures of gods and heroes.

Geometric patterns of inlaid silver

Decorative knob

Iron rivets

AXES

Axes with long wooden handles were the most common Viking weapon. T-shaped axes were usually used for working wood (p. 43). But the example above is so richly decorated that it must have been a weapon – and a sign of prestige or power.

Hole for wooden handle, which has rotted away

Rounded pommel

Broad iron blade

Iron axehead from Fyrkat, Denmark

Iron axehead from Trelleborg, Denmark

Double-edged sword from Bjørnsholm, Søndersø, Denmark

Hilt decorated with geometric patterns of silver and brass

DOUBLE-EDGED SWORDS

Swords were usually double-edged. The blacksmith (pp. 42–43) sometimes pattern-welded the blades for extra strength. He did this by fusing several strips of iron together. Then he twisted the metal, hammered it out, and polished it smooth. By adding carbon to the iron while it was red-hot, he produced sharp steel edges. Hilts and pommels were often highly decorated.

Pattern-welded iron blade

CHAIN GANG

In this detail from the Bayeux Tapestry (p. 10), Norman warriors carry weapons and chain-mail suits to their ships. The suits of mail (p. 13) are so heavy that each one is carried on a pole between two men. This also stops the chain-mail from getting tangled up. Viking weapons would have been similar.

Straight guard

Grip

Pommel

Iron sword from Denmark

Fuller, a central groove that makes the sword lighter and more flexible

15

Terrorizing the West

THE VIKINGS SWEPT into western Europe, terrorizing towns along the coast, plundering churches and grabbing riches, slaves, and land. The first recorded raid, on the famous monastery of Lindisfarne in 793, shocked the whole Christian world. From then on, attacks all over Europe intensified. Bands of Viking warriors roamed the North Sea and the English Channel, raiding choice targets at will. Soon the Vikings were venturing further inland. They sailed up the great rivers of Europe – the Rhine, Seine, Rhone, and Loire – and even overran Paris. The raiders began to spend the winters in areas they had captured. Then they set up bases to attack other targets. The Vikings often demanded huge payments for leaving an area in peace. Some warriors were off raiding for years. Björn Jarnsmiða and his companion Hasting spent three years with 62 ships in Spain, North Africa, France, and Italy. They lost a lot of their treasure in storms on the way home.

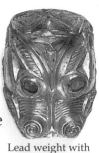

Lead weight with animal head made in Ireland

THROWN INTO THE THAMES
This Viking sword was found in the River Thames in London. This big English city was attacked many times, once by 94 ships. But it was never taken.

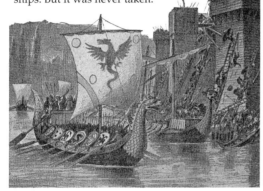

SOUVENIR OF PARIS
Paris was conquered on Easter Sunday, 28 March 845. Charles the Bald, the French king, had to pay the raiders 3,150 kg (7,000 lb) of silver to get peace. The Viking leader Ragnar even took a bar from the city gate as a souvenir. But he and most of his men died of disease on their way back to Scandinavia.

Rusted iron blade

HOLY SLAUGHTER
Lindisfarne is a small island off the east coast of England. The celebrated monastery there was destroyed by Vikings in 793. These warriors on a stone from the island may well be the Viking raiders. The *Anglo-Saxon Chronicle*, a contemporary English historical record, reported: "the ravages of heathen men miserably destroyed God's church on Lindisfarne, with plunder and slaughter."

RAIDING FRANCE
This picture of a Viking ship is in a French manuscript from around 1100. Viking ships attacked French towns and monasteries all through the 9th century. One group of Vikings settled in the Seine region. Another band under the chieftain Rollo made their homes around Rouen. This area became known as Normandy, "Land of the Northmen" (p. 10).

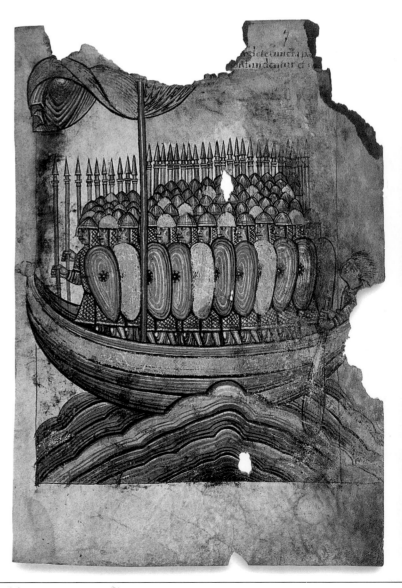

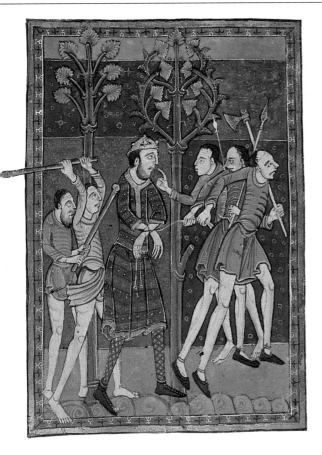

KILLING THE KING

King Edmund was king of East Anglia in England in 869. This 12th-century manuscript shows him being beaten by Vikings. Then they tied him to a tree and shot him full of arrows. He still refused to give up his belief in Christ, so they cut his head off. The Vikings later settled in East Anglia under their leader King Guthrum.

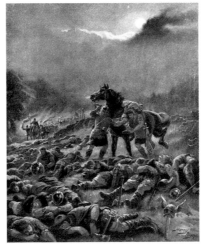

SCOTCHED

This is an imaginary scene from the Viking invasion of Scotland. Many of the raiders were Norwegians who came via the Shetland and Orkney Islands. From these resting places, the many Hebridean islands, the Isle of Man (pp. 37, 51), and Ireland were all within easy reach.

Interlace designs, typical of Dublin Viking art

IRISH CROOK

Raids on Ireland began in 795. By the 820s the Vikings had worked their way around the entire island. The town of Dublin became a thriving Viking trading centre with links to many other countries. This wooden animal head comes from a crook or walking stick. It was made in Dublin, but it is decorated in the Viking Ringerike style. It dates from early in the 11th century.

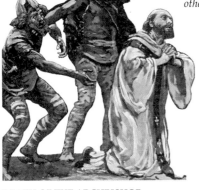

DEATH OF THE ARCHBISHOP

In 1011 Archbishop Alphege of Canterbury was seized by Vikings who were raiding the English countryside. They were angry because the English King Ethelred hadn't paid them fast enough. The archbishop refused to be ransomed. The Vikings, who were very drunk, pelted him with bones and the skulls of cattle. He was finally killed with a battle-axe.

RANVAIK'S SHRINE

This shrine or casket was made in Scotland or Ireland in the 8th century. It holds holy Christian relics. It was probably taken to Norway as loot. There the new owner inscribed a message in runes (pp. 58–59) on the bottom: "Ranvaik owns this casket".

Hollow box of yew wood covered in plates of tin and copper mixed with other metals

Small pieces of red enamel

Whole casket is shaped like a house

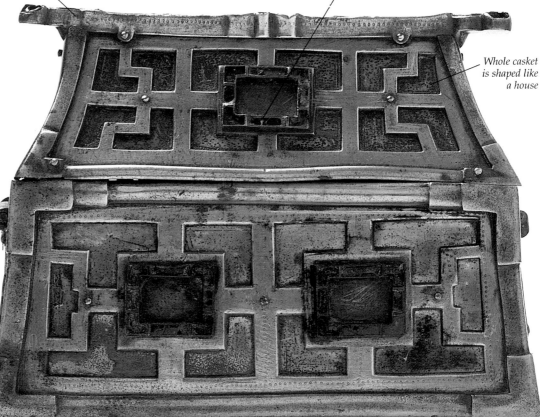

East into Russia

A SHORT SAIL ACROSS THE BALTIC SEA is all that separates Scandinavia from the rivers of Russia. Viking warriors and traders sailed into the Dniepr and Volga rivers and followed them all the way to the Black and Caspian Seas. From there, the great and mysterious cities of Constantinople (heart of the Byzantine empire) and Baghdad (capital of the Islamic Caliphate) were within easy reach. The history of Viking raids in the East is not as well recorded as in Western Europe. But all through Russia and beyond, Vikings left brooches, weapons, and runic inscriptions as traces of their travels. Traders swapped Siberian furs for silk, spices, and Arab silver. Viking warriors were even hired as Imperial guards in Constantinople.

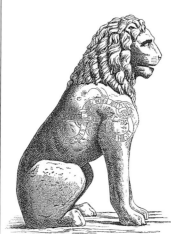

VIKING GRAFFITI
This stone lion once stood in the Greek port of Piraeus. A Viking traveller inscribed it with long looping bands of runes, the Scandinavian writing (pp. 58–59). Such graffiti is often the only evidence of where Vikings travelled. Much later, in 1687, Venetian soldiers carried the lion off to Venice. The runes have eroded too much to be read today.

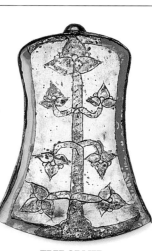

TREE OF LIFE
An Oriental tree of life is etched on the surface of this silver locket. It may have been an amulet, perhaps full of strong-smelling spices. The locket was found in a grave in Birka, Sweden. But it was probably made in the Volga area of Russia, or even as far south as Baghdad.

Silver loop for chain

EASTERN FASHIONS
Gotland is an island in the Baltic Sea. Gotland Vikings travelled far into Russia, and their excellent craftsmen often adopted styles from the east. These beads and pendant are made of rock-crystal set in silver. They were probably made in Gotland, where they were found. But the style is distinctly Slav or Russian.

High-quality rock crystal shaped like a convex lens

CHEQUERED PAST
This silver cup was made in the Byzantine empire in the 11th century. It was taken back to Gotland by Vikings, who added a name and a magical inscription on the bottom in runes. The cup was buried around 1361, and found by ditch-diggers in 1881.

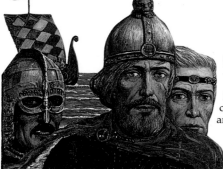

SWEDISH VIKINGS
Most of the Vikings who travelled to Russia and the east were Swedish. Of more than 85,000 Arab coins found in Scandinavia, 80,000 were found in Sweden. Many 11th-century Swedish rune stones tell of voyages to the south and east. They record the deaths of travellers in Russia, Greece, the Byzantine empire, and even Muslim lands. Most Viking settlements were temporary trading stations. Others, like Kiev and Novgorod, were more permanent. A sign of this is that women lived there too.

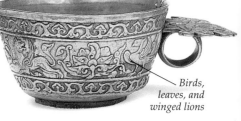

Birds, leaves, and winged lions

Fur hat

Fighting axe with
long wooden handle

Long knife in
leather sheath

Woollen tunic with
embroidered border

Baggy
trousers in
eastern
fashion

Knee-high
leather boots

Wooden
shield

Sword

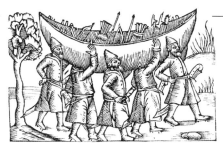

GOING OVERLAND
The Russian rivers were full of
rocks and rapids. The Vikings
dragged or carried their light
boats around these dangers.
Not everyone made it. Swedish
memorial stones record the
deaths of many travellers in
Russia and lands beyond.

A WELL-ARMED RUS
In the east, Vikings were called "Rus" by the local people.
This may be where the word Russia comes from. Arab writers
describe Viking traders armed with swords and carrying furs
of black fox and beaver. The Arab Ibn Fadhlan (p. 47, 55)
said the Rus he met in 922 were "the filthiest of God's
creatures". He noted with disgust that they all washed
in the same bowl of water, rinsing their hair, blowing
their noses, and spitting in it before passing
it on to someone else!

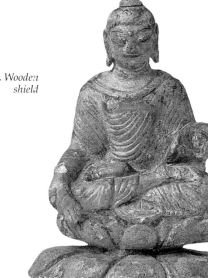

A VIKING BUDDHA?
Made in northern India in the 6th or 7th century,
this bronze Buddha found its way to the Viking
trading centre of Helgö in Sweden. It probably
stood in someone's house as a treasure.

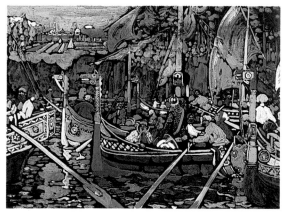

SONG OF THE VOLGA
This is *Song of the Volga* by the Russian painter Wassili
Kandinsky (1866–1944). The River Volga flows across
Russia all the way to the Caspian Sea. Viking traders sailed
up it in ships heavy with Arab silver. They had to pay taxes
to the Bulgars and Khazars who lived along its banks.

19

Discovering new lands

THE VIKINGS WERE DARING EXPLORERS. In search of new land, they sailed their slender ships into the frozen, uncharted waters of the North Atlantic. Most of the explorers came from Norway, where the valleys were crowded and farmland was scarce. They discovered the Faroe Islands, Iceland, and far-off Greenland and "Vinland" (America). As reports of these exciting discoveries got back to Scandinavia, ships full of eager settlers set sail. Between 870 and 930, for example, more than 10,000 Vikings arrived in Iceland. They found empty spaces, wild forests, and seas teeming with fish. The sea voyages were long and dangerous, and many ships were lost in storms. But the urge to travel to new lands was never dimmed.

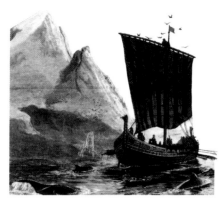

GREEN AND RED
A man called Gunnbjörn found Greenland after his ship was blown off course in a storm. The huge island was explored in 984 and 985 by Erik the Red, a chief who had been accused of murder and forced to leave Iceland. Erik encouraged hundreds of Icelanders to settle in Greenland.

THE THINGVELLIR
Iceland is a volcanic island. This high plain surrounded by great cliffs of lava was chosen as the site for the Althing, the governing assembly which met once a year in the open air (p. 29). It is thought to have first met in 930.

Iceland

Iceland was discovered in 870. In good weather it took seven days to get there from Norway. The first settler was Ingolf, from Sunnfjord, Norway. He built a large farm on a bay overlooking the sea. This later became the capital, Reykjavik. The settlers raised sheep, and used local iron and soapstone to make weapons and cooking pots. Soon they were exporting these natural resources, along with woollen and linen cloth.

REINDEER KILLS REINDEER
These arrowheads from Greenland are carved from reindeer antler. Iron was very scarce, so weapons had to be made from the materials at hand. Reindeer were a major source of food, and the settlers may have used these arrows to hunt them.

West Fjords

Faxa Fjord

Reykjavik

Thingvellir (Thing Plain)

Mt Hekla (volcano)

Vatna Jökull (huge glacier)

FIRE AND ICE LAND
Iceland's interior is harsh and inhospitable, with jagged mountains, glaciers, and several active volcanoes. But the coast is green and fertile. In the Viking Age there were also extensive forests between the mountains and the sea. By A.D. 930 the coast was densely populated. The interior was never really inhabited.

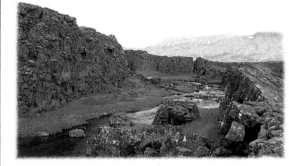

HELGE'S ANIMALS
This elegant piece of carved wood was discovered in the ruins of a house in Greenland. It dates from the 11th century. It may be the arm of a chair, or a tiller used to steer a boat (pp. 9, 11). The surface is carved with animals with big eyes that look like cats. A runic inscription at the end probably proclaims the owner's name, Helge.

America

Leif the Lucky, Erik the Red's son, also discovered land by accident when his ships went off course on a trip to Greenland. Around the year 1001, he became the first European to set foot on North America, probably in Newfoundland, Canada. He called it Vinland, "Wine Land". This strange name may come from giant huckleberries that Leif thought were red grapes. The Vikings also discovered Markland (Wood Land) and Helluland (Rock Land). These may be Labrador and Baffin Island to the north.

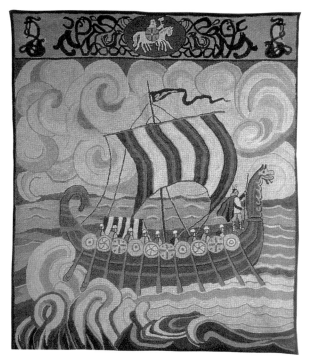
Modern tapestry showing Leif the Lucky sighting Vinland

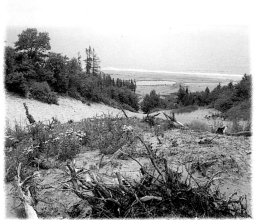
VIKINGS IN VINLAND
Only one Viking settlement has been found in North America. This is at L'Anse aux Meadows in Newfoundland. Large houses with thick turf walls have been unearthed. Only two Viking objects, a dress pin and a spindle whorl (p. 44), have turned up. Despite the fertile land and mild climate, the Viking settlements didn't last long. They were a long way from home, and the local people were hostile.

EXPLORING THE FROZEN NORTH
This rune stone was found at Kingiktorsuak, Greenland, at latitude 73° North. It proves that settlers explored the frozen north of the island. The stone was carved around the year 1300. Some time after this date, the last descendants of the Vikings in Greenland perished.

GREENLAND INUIT
The Inuit (Eskimos) made everything they needed from the natural resources of the land and sea. But the Vikings had to import timber, iron, and corn to survive.

Greenland

Most of this inhospitable island is covered in ice and snow. Erik the Red called it "Greenland" to encourage people to move there. The Vikings made two settlements, the eastern and western settlements, in the only areas where the land could be farmed. They built their farms on the edges of fjords, often far inland. They farmed sheep and cattle, but depended mainly on reindeer and seals for food.

WHALEBONE AXE
The Inuit in Greenland made weapons from the bones of seals, whales, and reindeer. This whalebone axehead from a Viking farm shows that the Vikings did the same. Its shape is very similar to iron axeheads (p. 15), but it wouldn't have been as strong. It is probably a toy made for a child.

Animal head

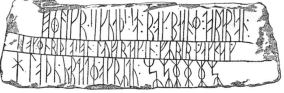

Animal with gaping jaws and huge teeth

A Viking fort

THE VIKINGS BUILT FOUR great circular forts in Denmark. Two of them, at Aggersborg and Fyrkat, are on the Jutland peninsula. The other two are at Trelleborg on the island of Sjælland and Nonnebakken on the island of Fyn. It used to be thought that King Svein Forkbeard built them as military camps for launching his invasion of England in 1013. But dendrochronology – tree-ring dating – has proved that the forts were built earlier, around 980. It is now thought that King Harald Bluetooth had them constructed to unify his kingdom and strengthen his rule. Bones dug up in cemeteries outside the ramparts prove that women and children lived there as well as men. Some of the fort buildings were workshops, where smiths forged weapons and jewellery from gold, silver, and iron.

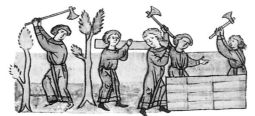

THE WALLS GO UP
The first step in building a fort was clearing the land and preparing the timber. This detail from a 15th-century Byzantine manuscript shows Swedish Vikings making the walls of Novgorod in Russia in the 10th century.

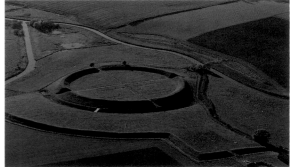

Aerial photograph of the site of the Trelleborg fortress

TRELLEBORG, FROM THE AIR
The forts had a strict geometrical layout. Each one lay within a high circular rampart, a mound of earth and turf held up by a wooden framework. This was divided into four quadrants by two roads, one running north–south, the other east–west. Four long houses sat in a square in each of the quadrants. The roads were paved with timber. Covered gateways, which may have been topped with towers, guarded the spots where the roads met the rampart. The largest fort, Aggersborg, was 240 m (790 ft) in diameter. Trelleborg was much smaller, 136 m (445 ft) across. Trelleborg is unusual because 15 extra houses were built outside the main fort. These were protected by their own rampart. All four forts were built on important land routes, possibly so that Harald could keep an eye on the area in case of rebellion.

Two roads criss-crossing fort

River

Cemetery

Houses

Circular ramparts built of earth and turf and faced with wood

Extra outer rampart

Ditch

Four houses around a square yard

Layout of the Trelleborg fortress

TRELLEBORG HOUSE, SIDE VIEW
The buildings at the forts were made of wood, which rotted away a long time ago. All that is left are ghostly outlines and black holes where the posts once stood. This replica of a house was built in 1948. It is 29.4 m (96 ft 5 in) long. The elegant curving roof is "hog-backed" in shape. House-shaped gravestones and caskets from England give an idea of how it once looked. Experts now believe that there was only one roof, which reached all the way down to the short outer posts.

Iron blade, badly rusted now

Silver inlaid in geometric patterns

Gables decorated with projections called finials

THE COMPLETE WORKS OF HARALD BLUETOOTH
The four forts were only one of King Harald Bluetooth's huge projects, which have changed the Danish landscape to this day. His engineering works include the first bridge in Scandinavia, a huge wooden structure at Ravning Enge in Jutland. He also strengthened the Danevirke, a massive wall that protected Denmark from invasion from the south. And he built a grand memorial at Jelling in Jutland (above). This includes the Jelling Stone, the biggest and grandest of Viking memorial stones (pp. 60–61).

GUARDING THE FORT
Various weapons have been found at the forts. This beautiful T-shaped axehead (p. 15) comes from a grave at Trelleborg. It was probably a symbol of power, not a working weapon. A light throwing spear was found in a guardhouse at the Fyrkat fortress.

TRELLEBORG HOUSE, FRONT VIEW
The houses were built of upright staves (wooden planks) set straight into the earth. They all followed a standard pattern. The main door at each end opened into a small room. These led in turn into a huge central living room, where a big fire always burned. Farmhouses like the ones excavated at Vorbasse in Jutland have a similar layout. The wood must have rotted quickly, and there is no evidence of repairs. The forts were probably only inhabited for a few years. King Harald was forced into exile in 986. Soon after this date, the forts he had built were left to rot.

Sturdy wooden posts hold up roof

Walls made of staves (planks)

Main door

Smoke hole over fire that burned in a hearth in the middle of the central living room

Roof is covered in overlapping shingles (wooden tiles)

Finials

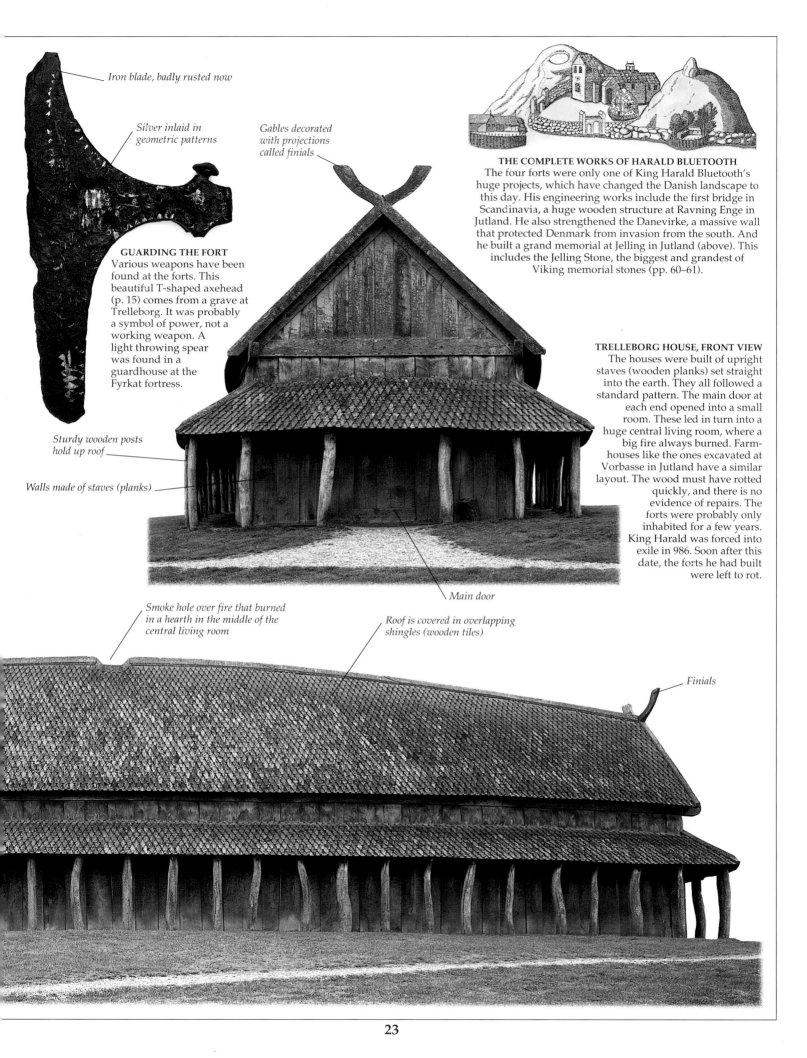

Other ships

THE VIKINGS BUILT SHIPS and boats of many shapes and sizes, suited to different waters and uses. They were all variations on the same design, with overlapping strakes (planks), a keel, and matching prow and stern. Only the longest, fastest vessels were taken raiding. Cargo ships were slower and fatter, with lots of room for storing goods. Other boats were specially made for sailing in narrow inlets and rivers, following the coast, or for crossing oceans. There were fishing boats, ferries for carrying passengers across rivers and fjords, and small boats designed to ply lakes. Small rowing boats were also carried on board larger boats.

BRONZE AGE BOATS
Rock carvings in Sweden and Norway show boats from as early as 1800 B.C. Sails were developed in Scandinavia just before the Viking Age, around A.D. 700. Before then, all ships were rowed.

LEIF SIGHTS AMERICA
Explorers sailed wide-bodied, sturdy ships. These were much heavier than warships and had more space for passengers and their belongings and supplies. In this dramatic interpretation of Leif the Lucky's voyage to America (p. 21), Leif is shown pointing in wonder at the new continent. His other hand holds the tiller. The raised deck at the stern (back) can be clearly seen. Leif was Erik the Red's son (p. 20), and is also known as Leif Eriksson.

ROWING BOAT
Rowing boats were made just like miniature ships. This is a replica of one of the three small rowing boats buried with the Gokstad ship (pp. 8–9). It had two pairs of slender oars and a stubby steering oar.

Steering oar

Two sets of oars

CARGO SHIP
This is the prow of one of the five ships from Roskilde Fjord, Denmark (pp. 10–11). It is a merchant ship, 13.8 m (45 ft 3 in) long and 3.3 m (10 ft 10 in) wide and probably made locally. It could carry five tonnes of cargo. This was stowed in the middle of the ship and covered with animal hides to protect it from the rain. The crew could still steer and work the sail from decks at the prow and stern. The ship may have belonged to a merchant who sailed along the coast to Norway to pick up iron and soapstone and across the Baltic Sea in search of luxuries like amber.

Hole for rope

Forward oarport (hole for oar)

Gunwale, top strake

A copy of the prow (below) in place

Overlapping strakes held together with iron nails or clench-bolts

ONE-PIECE
The cargo ship above is put together with great skill. The shipbuilder carved the entire prow from a single piece of oak. The keel was made first. Then the prow and stern were nailed to the keel. Finally the strakes and deck boards were fitted.

The lines of the strakes are continued in elegant carvings on the prow

DROPPING ANCHOR
Every ship needs an anchor. The anchor of the Oseberg ship (pp. 54–57) was solid iron with an oak frame. It weighed 10 kg (22 lb). This stone anchor comes from Iceland.

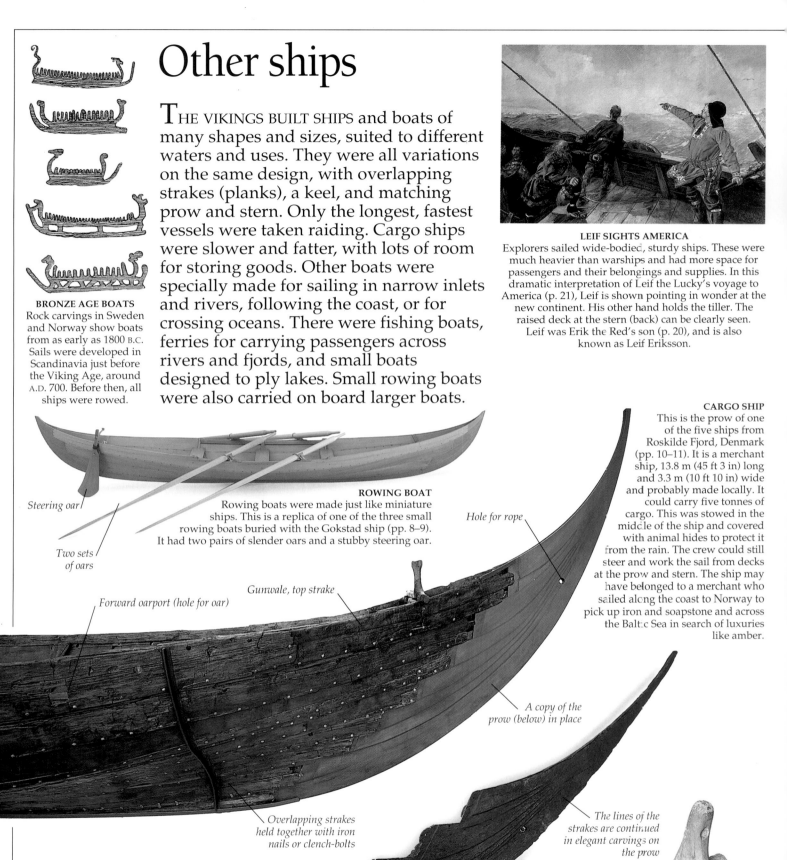

ROAR EGE, FRONT VIEW

Named *Roar Ege*, this is a replica of the merchant ship from Roskilde on the opposite page. It was specially built to see how much cargo the ship could hold and how many men were needed to sail it. The ship has oars, but the crew of four to six only use them for manoeuvring in tight spots. Usually they rely on a large sail. In good winds, *Roar Ege* averages 4 knots (7.5 km/h), and has reached a speed of 8 knots (15 km/h). The ship was ideally suited to sailing in the Baltic Sea and Danish coastal waters. The original may have been taken up rivers or into the North Sea.

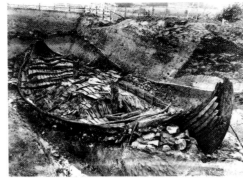

THE OSEBERG SHIP

One of the most beautiful Viking vessels is the Oseberg ship (pp. 54–57). It was not as sturdy as the Gokstad ship, and was probably built to cruise coastal waters. This is a scene from the ship's excavation.

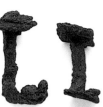

RIVETING STUFF
Iron rivets held the strakes together. Often they are all that is left of a ship once the wood has rotted away.

High prow, which stops ship from nose-diving in rough water

Mooring post

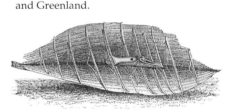

SETTLERS' VESSEL
This is a model of a sturdy cargo ship with a square sail and shrouds (ropes) securing the mast. Ships like this carried settlers to Iceland and Greenland.

Each side has three oarports, two near the prow and one at the stern

Pronounced keel, needed for sailing

Sternpost, almost identical to prow or stempost

OUT OF TUNE
The remains of another large ship were found at Tune, across the Oslo Fjord from the Gokstad and Oseberg ship mounds. The Tune ship is built of oak, with a pine steering oar and cross-beams. It was about 20 m (66 ft) long, a little shorter than the Gokstad ship.

INSIDE *ROAR EGE*

This view inside the stern shows how Viking ships were made. The hull was built first. This was then strengthened with cross-beams secured to the strakes with curved "knees". The top layer of cross-beams could support decks or rowing benches.

Hull, made of eight strakes

Knee

Top of two levels of cross-beams

Stringer, a horizontal strengthener

Stern oarport

Trading east and west

THE VIKINGS WERE GREAT TRADERS who travelled far beyond Scandinavia buying and selling goods. The riches of the north included timber for ship-building; iron for making tools and weapons; furs for warm clothing; skins from whales and seals for ship ropes; and whale bones and walrus ivory for carving. These were carried to far-flung places and exchanged for local goods. The traders returned from Britain with wheat, silver, and cloth, and brought wine, salt, pottery, and gold back from the Mediterranean. They sailed across the Baltic Sea and upriver into Russia, then continued on foot or camel as far as Constantinople (now Istanbul) and Jerusalem. In markets all along the way, they haggled over the price of glass, exotic spices, silks, and slaves. Markets and towns grew as centres for trade. Big Viking market towns included Birka in Sweden, Kaupang in Norway, Hedeby in Denmark, York in England, Dublin in Ireland, and Kiev in Ukraine.

THE SLAVE TRADE
Some Vikings made their fortune trading slaves. They took many Christian prisoners, like this 9th-century French monk. Some slaves were taken home for heavy farm and building work. Others were sold for silver to Arab countries.

Coin and die for striking (making) coins, from York, England

Three early Danish coins

THE COMING OF COINS
Coins only became common towards the end of the Viking Age. Before then, goods were usually bought with pieces of silver or bartered – swapped for items of similar value. The first Danish coins were struck in the 9th century. But it wasn't until 975, under King Harald Bluetooth, that coins were made in large numbers.

Brass Buddha-like figure

Colourful enamel

Bands of brass

MADE IN ENGLAND?
One of the many beautiful objects found with the Oseberg ship (pp. 54–57) was the mysterious "Buddha bucket". Its handle is attached to two brass figures with crossed legs that look just like Buddhas. But the Vikings were not Buddhists, and the craftsmanship suggests that the figures were made in England. So how did the splendid bucket end up in a queen's grave in Norway? It must have been traded and brought back from England.

Staves (strips) of yew wood

RHINE GLASS
Only rich Vikings drank from glass cups. Many have been found in Swedish graves. This glass must have been bought or stolen in the Rhineland, in modern Germany.

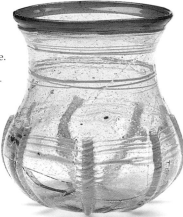

TUSK, TUSK
The Vikings hunted walruses for their hide, which was turned into ship ropes. The large animals were skinned in a spiral, starting from the tail. Traders also sold the animal's ivory tusks, either unworked or beautifully carved.

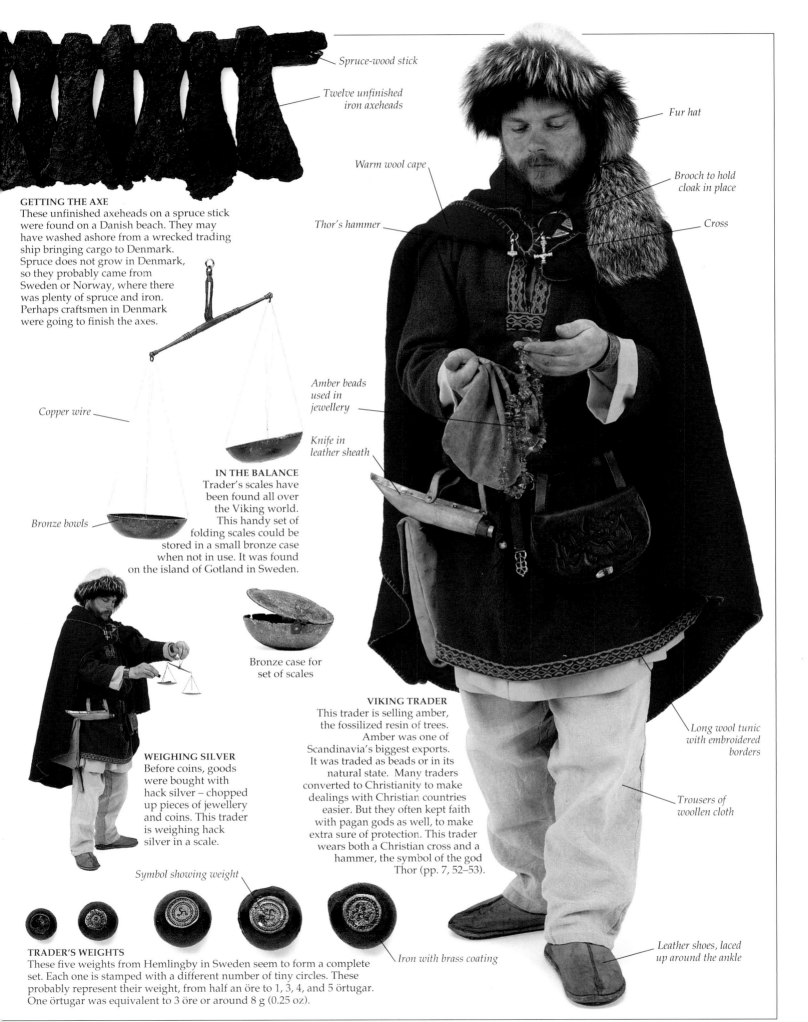

Spruce-wood stick

Twelve unfinished
iron axeheads

Fur hat

Warm wool cape

Brooch to hold
cloak in place

Thor's hammer

Cross

GETTING THE AXE

These unfinished axeheads on a spruce stick
were found on a Danish beach. They may
have washed ashore from a wrecked trading
ship bringing cargo to Denmark.
Spruce does not grow in Denmark,
so they probably came from
Sweden or Norway, where there
was plenty of spruce and iron.
Perhaps craftsmen in Denmark
were going to finish the axes.

Amber beads
used in
jewellery

Copper wire

Knife in
leather sheath

IN THE BALANCE

Trader's scales have
been found all over
the Viking world.
This handy set of
folding scales could be
stored in a small bronze case
when not in use. It was found
on the island of Gotland in Sweden.

Bronze bowls

Bronze case for
set of scales

WEIGHING SILVER

Before coins, goods
were bought with
hack silver – chopped
up pieces of jewellery
and coins. This trader
is weighing hack
silver in a scale.

VIKING TRADER

This trader is selling amber,
the fossilized resin of trees.
Amber was one of
Scandinavia's biggest exports.
It was traded as beads or in its
natural state. Many traders
converted to Christianity to make
dealings with Christian countries
easier. But they often kept faith
with pagan gods as well, to make
extra sure of protection. This trader
wears both a Christian cross and a
hammer, the symbol of the god
Thor (pp. 7, 52–53).

Long wool tunic
with embroidered
borders

Trousers of
woollen cloth

Symbol showing weight

TRADER'S WEIGHTS

These five weights from Hemlingby in Sweden seem to form a complete
set. Each one is stamped with a different number of tiny circles. These
probably represent their weight, from half an öre to 1, 3, 4, and 5 örtugar.
One örtugar was equivalent to 3 öre or around 8 g (0.25 oz).

Iron with brass coating

Leather shoes, laced
up around the ankle

Kings and freemen

VIKING SOCIETY HAD THREE CLASSES – slaves, freemen, and nobles. Most of the hard labour was done by slaves, or *thralls*. Many were foreigners captured in war (p. 26). Wealthy people sometimes had their slaves killed and buried with them. Slaves could be freed. Freemen included farmers, traders, craftsmen, warriors, and big landowners. At the beginning of the Viking Age, there were many local chieftains (nobles) who ruled over small areas. They were subject to the rule of the Thing, the local assembly where all freemen could voice their opinions and complain about others. But chieftains and kings gradually increased their wealth and power by raiding and conquering foreign lands. By the end of the Viking Age, around A.D. 1050, Norway, Denmark, and Sweden were each ruled by a single, powerful king, and the role of the Things had declined.

WELL-GROOMED
The well-off Viking warrior or chieftain took pride in his appearance. This Viking carved from elk antler has neatly trimmed hair and beard.

PEASANT WARRIOR
This peasant was not rich, and dressed simply. But he was a freeman, and owned his own farm, which his wife would look after when he went to war. The 10th-century poem *Rigspula* describes a peasant couple. He makes furniture and his wife weaves. They have a son called Karl, which means farmer or free-man. Karl's wife wears fine goatskin and carries keys, a symbol of her status (p. 33).

Simple leather belt

Wooden axe-handle

Plain iron axehead

Wooden shield with iron boss

Plain woollen trousers

Toggle (fastener) made of antler

Goatskin

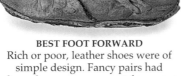

BEST FOOT FORWARD
Rich or poor, leather shoes were of simple design. Fancy pairs had coloured uppers, ornamental seams, or even inscriptions. The most common leather for shoes was goatskin.

Leather shoes

FIGHTING IT OUT
This is *Duel at Skiringsal*, painted by the Norwegian Johannes Flintoe in the 1830s. Disputes were often settled by a duel, which could end in death. These gruesome fights were forbidden by law in Iceland and Norway around the year 1000. Arguments could also be sorted out by the Thing or by "ordeals". In these, men would try to prove their innocence by walking over red-hot iron or picking stones from a cauldron of burning water. The Vikings believed that the gods would protect the innocent.

FANCY HAT
The rich wore expensive clothes and imported jewellery. These parts of an elaborate cap were made in Kiev in Ukraine and worn by a nobleman in Birka, Sweden.

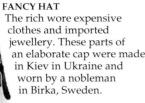

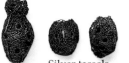

Silver cap mount

Silver tassels

Braids for fastening cloak

Wool tunic embroidered with animals and faces

TO CAP IT OFF
This silk cap was worn by a rich man or woman in the Viking town of York, England. The silk may have been imported from faraway Constantinople.

Cloak embroidered with human faces

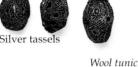

Bronze brooch for holding cloak in place

Tunic was often worn over linen undershirt

Dyed woollen trousers

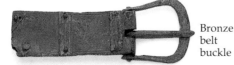

Bronze belt buckle

BROOCHES AND BUCKLES
All Viking men wore brooches and buckles to fasten their clothes. But the richer they were, the more ornate their brooch or buckle. These ones come from Gotland, Sweden.

MAMMEN CHIEFTAIN
Fine clothes, tablecloths, white bread, and silver cups were all signs of nobility. This man is wearing a reconstruction of clothes found in a nobleman's grave in Mammen, Denmark. They are made of high-quality wool and silk, decorated with embroidered borders and even gold and silver thread. The noble couple in the poem *Rigspula* have a son called Iarl, which means earl. He owns land, rides horses, and can read and write runes (pp. 58–59). His wife Erna is slender and wise. Their youngest child is called Konr ungr, which means king.

Cloak of dyed wool with embroidered borders

BORDER FACES
The border of the Mammen cloak was a panel of silk embroidered with human faces. No one knows who the faces are. But the silk was imported, and the beautiful decoration shows how wealthy the man was.

Fur trim

THINGS AND ALTHINGS
Each district had its own assembly, or Thing. Meetings were held outdoors at a special spot. This is a 19th-century painting of the Icelandic Althing, held once a year (p. 20). One observer said that "Icelanders have no king, only the law".

Women and children

Viking women were independent. While the men were away on expeditions, women ran households and farms. A woman could choose her own husband, and could sue for divorce if he beat her or was unfaithful. On runestones (pp. 58–59), women were praised for their good housekeeping or skill in handiwork such as embroidery. Wealthy women raised runestones and paid for bridges to be built. Viking children didn't go to school. Instead they worked in the fields and workshops, and helped with cooking, spinning, and weaving. Not all women and children stayed home. Many joined their husbands or fathers in colonies such as England. They hid somewhere safe during battles, and came out later to help set up new villages.

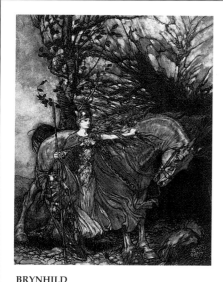

BRYNHILD
This is a romantic engraving of Brynhild. According to legend, she was a Valkyrie, a woman warrior (p. 53). In reality, there is no evidence that any Viking women were warriors, or even traders or craftsworkers. But one female scald (poet) and a female rune carver are known.

TOY HORSE
About 900 years ago, a small boy or girl in Trondheim, Norway, played with this toy horse made of wood. Children also had toy boats. They played board games and made music with small pipes (p. 50). In the summer young Vikings swam and played ball; in the winter they skated and played in the snow.

Two carved animal heads with open jaws

BONE SMOOTH
One of a woman's main responsibilities was making clothes for the whole family (pp. 44–45). After she had woven a piece of linen, a woman probably stretched it across a smoothing board and rubbed it with a glass ball until it was smooth and shiny. This board from Norway is made of whalebone.

Piece of leather covers point, so boys will not hurt each other

Toy spear made of wood

Woollen tunic with embroidered collar

STARTING YOUNG
Viking boys played with toy weapons made of wood. They probably began serious weapon practice in their early teens. Some young men seem to have gone raiding when they were as young as sixteen.

Leather bag

Decorated belt end

Toy sword

Antler, probably from an elk

Linen head-dress tied
under the chin

WELL COMBED
Combs carved out of bone or antler
have been found all over the Viking
world. These two are from Birka in Sweden.
Viking men and women made sure their hair was well
combed. They also used metal tweezers
to pluck out unwanted hairs, and tiny
metal ear scoops to clean out their ears.

Iron rivets

Oval brooches

DAILY DRESS
Viking women were very particular about
their appearance. This woman is wearing a
long under-dress. On top she has a short
over-dress, like a pinafore dress. This is
held up by two oval brooches.
An Arab who visited the town of
Hedeby around A.D. 950 said that
Viking women wore make-up
around their eyes to increase
their beauty. He also noted
that many men did the same.

Hair tied in bun

Drinking
horn

DRESS
FASTENERS
Oval brooches were only worn
by women. This pair comes from Ågerup in
Denmark. Finding such brooches in a grave shows
that the dead person was a woman. Although the
cloth of the dress has usually rotted away, the
position of the brooches on the shoulders shows
how they were worn.

Child's tunic

Train of dress

SWEDISH WOMAN
This silver pendant is from
Birka, Sweden. It is in the
shape of a woman in a dress
with a triangular train. She is
carrying a drinking horn, and
may be a Valkyrie (p. 53).

Child's shoes

Knotted
hairstyle

Bead necklace

Large ring
brooch

ALL DRESSED UP
Like the one above, this
small pendant shows a
well-dressed woman. She is
wearing a shawl over a long,
flowing dress. Her hair is tied
in an elegant, knotted style.
Her beads and a large
brooch are easy to identify.
The importance of pendants
like these is unclear.
They could have had some
magical meaning.
The figures represented
may even be goddesses.

Shawl

Over-dress

Long under-
dress with
flowing train

Long under-dress

Over-dress decorated
with woven bands

At home

HOME LIFE REVOLVED around a central hall or living room. The lay-out was much the same all over the Viking world. A long, open hearth (fireplace) burned in the centre, with a smoke hole in the ceiling above. The floor was stamped earth. The people sat and slept on raised platforms along the curved walls. Pillows and cushions stuffed with duck down or chicken feathers made this more comfortable. Well-off homes might have a few bits of wooden furniture and a locked chest for precious belongings. Houses often had smaller rooms for cooking or spinning on either side of the main hall. Small buildings with low floors dug out of the ground were used as houses, workshops, weaving sheds, or animal barns. A chieftain's hall could be lined with wall hangings or carved or painted wooden panels. Around the year 1000, an Icelandic poet described panels decorated with scenes of gods and legends in the hall of a great chieftain. The poem was called *Húsdrápa*, which means "poem in praise of the house".

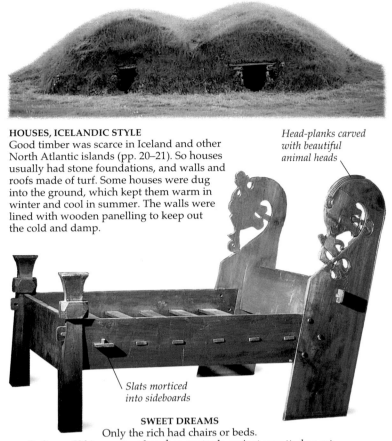

HOUSES, ICELANDIC STYLE
Good timber was scarce in Iceland and other North Atlantic islands (pp. 20–21). So houses usually had stone foundations, and walls and roofs made of turf. Some houses were dug into the ground, which kept them warm in winter and cool in summer. The walls were lined with wooden panelling to keep out the cold and damp.

Head-planks carved with beautiful animal heads

Slats morticed into sideboards

SWEET DREAMS
Only the rich had chairs or beds.
Ordinary Vikings sat on benches or stools, or just squatted or sat cross-legged on the floor. At night, they stretched out on rugs on the raised platforms. The wealthy woman in the Oseberg ship (pp. 54–57) was buried with not one, but three beds. This is a replica of the finest one. It is made of beech wood. The head-planks are carved in the form of animal heads with arching necks (p. 9). The woman probably slept on a feather mattress, and was kept warm by an eiderdown, a quilt filled with down or feathers.

Small window, a hole with no glass that may have had shutters

Turf roof was green with grass in summer, and covered with snow in winter

End view of Trondheim house

TRONDHEIM HOUSE
This is a model of a house built in Trondheim, Norway in the year 1003. Its walls are horizontal logs notched and fitted together at the corners. A layer of birchbark was laid on the pointed roof and covered in turf. The bark would have kept the water out, while the earth and grass acted as insulation. Houses were built in various other ways, depending on local traditions and the materials at hand. Wooden walls were often made of upright posts, or staves, as in the Danish forts (pp. 22–23). Others had walls of wattle (interwoven branches) smeared with daub (clay or dung) to make them waterproof. Roofs could be covered in shingles (wooden tiles), thatch, turf, or matted reeds.

Side view of Trondheim house

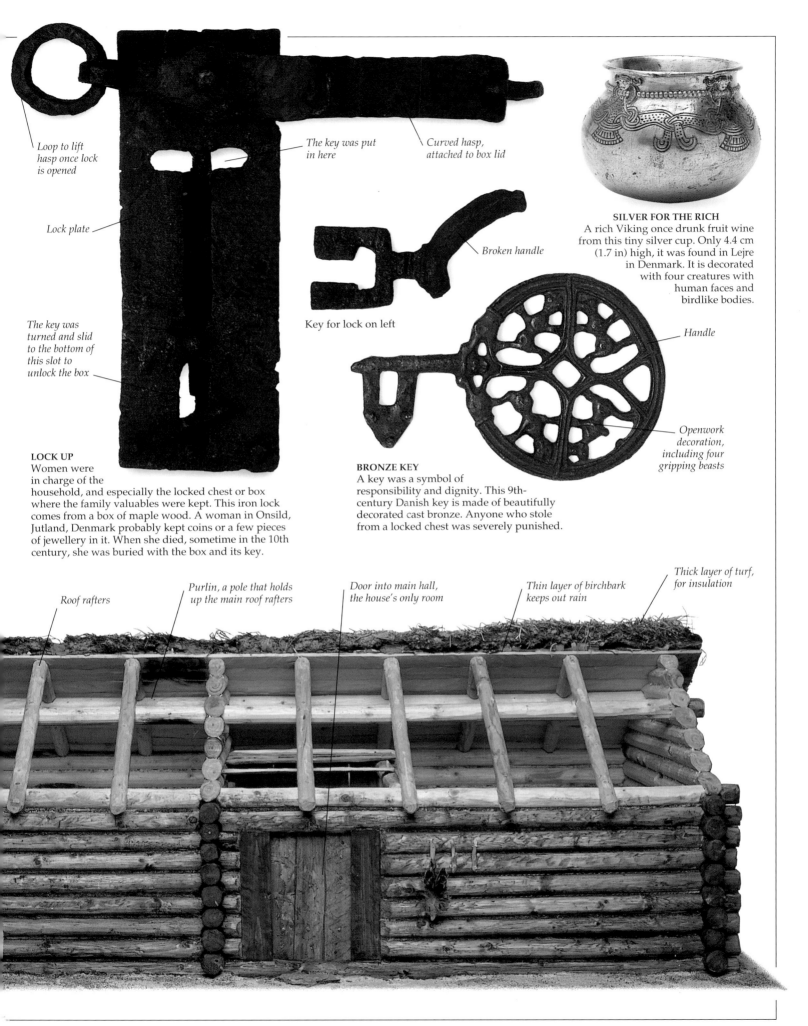

Loop to lift
hasp once lock
is opened

The key was put
in here

Curved hasp,
attached to box lid

Lock plate

SILVER FOR THE RICH
A rich Viking once drunk fruit wine
from this tiny silver cup. Only 4.4 cm
(1.7 in) high, it was found in Lejre
in Denmark. It is decorated
with four creatures with
human faces and
birdlike bodies.

Broken handle

The key was
turned and slid
to the bottom of
this slot to
unlock the box

Key for lock on left

Handle

LOCK UP
Women were
in charge of the
household, and especially the locked chest or box
where the family valuables were kept. This iron lock
comes from a box of maple wood. A woman in Onsild,
Jutland, Denmark probably kept coins or a few pieces
of jewellery in it. When she died, sometime in the 10th
century, she was buried with the box and its key.

BRONZE KEY
A key was a symbol of
responsibility and dignity. This 9th-
century Danish key is made of beautifully
decorated cast bronze. Anyone who stole
from a locked chest was severely punished.

Openwork
decoration,
including four
gripping beasts

Roof rafters

Purlin, a pole that holds
up the main roof rafters

Door into main hall,
the house's only room

Thin layer of birchbark
keeps out rain

Thick layer of turf,
for insulation

Meal time

ALL DAY LONG, the fire in the hearth was kept burning for cooking and heating. The hole in the roof above the fire didn't work very well, so Viking houses were always full of smoke. Rich households had baking ovens in separate rooms. These were heated by placing hot stones inside them. As darkness fell, work on the farm or in the workshop had to stop, and people would gather for the main meal of the day. The rich and the poor ate very different meals, served in different ways. For instance, most Vikings drank beer made from malted barley and hops. But while the poor drank from wooden mugs, the rich used drinking horns with fancy metal rims. They also enjoyed wine imported in barrels from Germany.

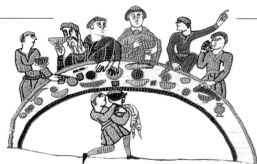

NORMAN FEAST
This feast scene from the Bayeux Tapestry (p. 10) shows a table laden with food and dishes. Vikings sat around trestle tables. The wealthy had richly decorated knives and spoons and imported pottery cups and jugs. More ordinary people ate and drank from wooden bowls and cups.

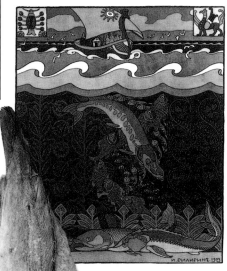

FOOD FROM THE SEA
The sea was full of fish. For Vikings who lived near the coast, fish was the staple food. The bones of cod, herring, and haddock have been found in many Viking settlements. People also caught eels and freshwater fish, such as trout, in the many rivers and lakes that criss-cross Scandinavia.

HOME GROWN
Cabbages (above) and peas were the most common vegetables. Many Vikings grew their own.

DRIED COD
Food had to be preserved so it would keep through the winter. Fish and meat were hung in the wind to dry. They could also be pickled in salt water. Salt was collected by boiling sea water, a boring job usually given to slaves. Fish and meat were probably also smoked.

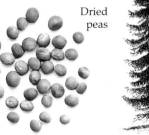

Dried peas

Pine tree, source of kernels and bark

PEAS AND PINE BARK
Poor Vikings made bread with whatever they could find. One loaf found in Sweden contained dried peas and pine bark.

Cumin, a spice found in the Oseberg burial

FIT FOR A QUEEN
Horseradish was one of the seasonings found in the Oseberg burial (pp. 54–57), along with wheat, oats, and fruit.

A Norman cook lifts chunks of cooked meat off a stove with a two-pronged fork.

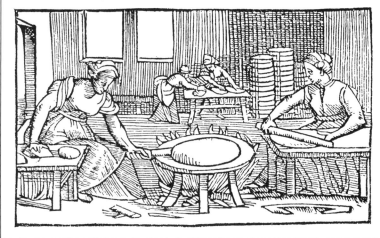

BAKING BREAD
Bread was kneaded in wooden troughs. Then it was baked on a griddle over a fire (as in this 16th-century Swedish picture) or in a pan that sat in the embers. Barley bread was most common, but rich people had loaves made of finer wheat flour.

POACHED EGGS
In the Atlantic Islands, Viking settlers gathered gulls' eggs for eating. They also roasted the gulls.

GARLIC BULB
Like modern cooks, the Vikings added garlic and onion to meat stews and soups.

A HARE IN MY SOUP
Hares were trapped and hunted. The Vikings also hunted elk, deer, bears, wild boars, reindeer, seals, and whales for meat. Sheep, cattle, pigs, goats, geese, chickens, turkeys, and even horses were raised to be eaten.

Suspension loop

COOKING CAULDRON
Food was prepared around the hearth in the centre of the living room. Meat was stewed in huge pots called cauldrons made of iron or soapstone. Some cauldrons were hung over the fire on a chain from the roof-beam. Others, like this one from the Oseberg ship, were supported by a tripod.

Iron handle

CAUGHT ON THE WING
Game birds like this duck were trapped or hunted with short arrows. Roasted on a spit, it would make a tasty meal.

One of the tripod's three legs

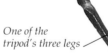
Blackberry

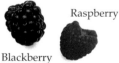
Raspberry

BERRY TASTY
Berries and wild fruits such as apples, cherries, and plums were gathered in the summer. Vikings may have grown fruit trees in gardens as well as picking fruit wild in the forest.

Old crack   *Repair holes*

The pronged feet were stuck into the earth floor to keep the cauldron stable

Iron cauldron

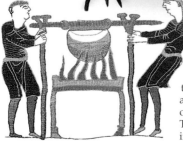

BAYEUX BARBECUE
In this scene from the Bayeux Tapestry (p. 10), two Norman cooks heat a cauldron. The fire sits in a tray like a barbecue. To the left, a third man lifts cooked chunks of meat off a stove onto a plate. The Vikings may have cooked in similar ways.

PATCHED
This clay cooking pot has four holes where a patch was stuck over a crack.

Animals, wild and imagined

BEARS, WOLVES, mink, foxes, deer, and wild boar all roamed the dark forests of Norway and Sweden. Whales, otters, seals, walruses, and reindeer lived in the far north. Sea birds flocked along the coasts, and game birds were common inland. The Vikings hunted most of these animals for their meat. They made clothes and bedding from feathers, furs, and hides, and bones and tusks were raw materials for jewellery, tools, and everyday objects like knife-handles. Many of the finest objects were then traded (pp. 26–27). Viking legends and art are also crammed with wild beasts. But the animals which decorate jewellery, tools, and weapons are not real. They have been turned into fantastic and acrobatic creatures. Their hips are spirals, and plant shoots spring from their bodies. Some beasts become ribbons that twist around each other in intricate patterns.

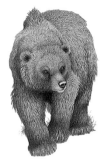

BROWN BEAR
Bears were hunted in the far north. Their skins were made into jackets and cloaks, and their claws and teeth were worn as pendants. Warriors may have thought that some of the bear's strength and courage would rub off on them (p. 14).

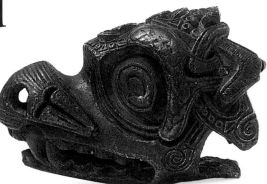

BRONZE BEAST
This fierce animal with snarling teeth comes from a horse's harness bow (p. 41). It may have been intended to scare enemies and protect the horse and wagon.

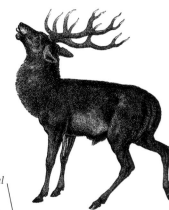

STAG
Elk, deer, and reindeer all have big antlers. Craftsmen sawed and carved these to create combs (pp. 31, 59). Deer skin was used for clothes and possibly wall and bed coverings. Venison (deer meat) was also dried or roasted, and eaten.

Gilt (gold-coated) silver

Owl

Bird of prey

BIRD BROOCH
This brooch was found in a woman's grave in Birka, Sweden. It once decorated a belt worn by someone living in Eastern Europe by the river Volga (pp. 18–19). A Viking took it home to Sweden, where a jeweller converted it into a brooch. The birds are quite realistic, and are easy to identify. A Viking craftsman would have turned them into fantastic creatures.

FANTASTIC ANIMAL
This brooch from Norway is in the shape of a slender, snake-like animal. It is caught up in a thin ribbon twisting in a fantastic pattern. This is known as the Urnes style of Viking art, after wood carvings on a church at Urnes in Norway.

Head of animal

Bronze, cast in a mould

This is an "openwork" brooch

GRIPPING BEAST

The acrobatic "gripping beast" became popular in Viking art in the 9th century. This playful animal writhes and turns inside out, gripping its own legs and even its throat.

Gripping beast from a 9th-century Danish brooch

Unlike deer, sheep do not shed their horns every year, so the horns get bigger with age

Each horn of an old Manx Loghtan ram (male) can weigh 350 g (12 oz) and reach 45 cm (1.5 ft) in length

SNAKE CHARM

Snakes were common in Viking lands, and are important in poems and sagas (p. 50–51). This silver snake pendant was worn by a Swedish woman as a good luck charm or amulet.

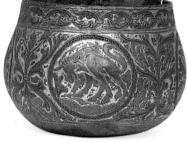

CAROLINGIAN CUP

Craftsmen in other areas based their decoration on real animals. This cup was made further south in the Carolingian empire, in modern France or Germany. It is made of gilt (gold-coated) silver decorated with the figure of a bull-like animal and symmetrical leaves of the acanthus plant. The cup must have been traded or plundered, because it was found in a Viking hoard at Halton Moor, England, with a silver neck-ring (p. 47) and a gold pendant (p. 46).

LONE WOLF

The wolf roamed wild in the mountains of Scandinavia. Then, as now, people were terrified of its eerie howl. In Viking legend, the god Odin is gobbled up by a monstrous wolf, Fenrir (p. 51). This is one of the horrible events of *Ragnarök*, the "Doom of the Gods".

HORNED HELMET

The Manx Loghtan sheep goes back to the Viking age. Now it is only found on the Isle of Man, an island between England and Ireland that was colonized by Vikings in the 9th century. Sheep were farmed all over the Viking world (pp. 38–39). In mountainous areas, Viking shepherds took their flocks to high pastures for the warm summer months. The Manx Loghtan sheep shed its wool naturally, so it didn't have to be sheared. It could grow two, four, or even six horns.

Farming

MOST VIKINGS WERE FARMERS. They often had to work infertile land in harsh weather. The difficult conditions led many farmers to set sail for faraway lands like Iceland (pp. 20–21), where they hoped to find fertile soil and more space for their animals and crops. Sheep, cows, pigs, goats, horses, poultry, and geese were all raised for eating. The milk of cattle, goats, and sheep was drunk or turned into butter and cheese. Farms often had separate byres, sheds where cattle could pass the winter. Even so, many died of cold or starvation. Rich farms had byres to house a hundred cattle. A man's wealth was often measured in animals. Othere, a merchant from northern Norway, told King Alfred of England that he had 20 cattle, 20 sheep, 20 pigs, and a herd of 600 reindeer. But his main source of income was the furs he traded.

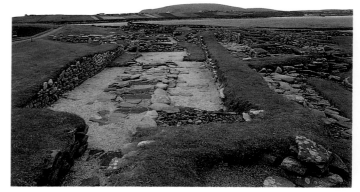

JARLSHOF FARM
The ruins of a 9th-century Viking farmhouse on the Shetland Islands. It had two rooms, a long hall and a kitchen. The farmers sat and slept on platforms that ran along the curved walls. A hearth burned in the centre of the hall.

SHEARS
Vikings sheared sheep, cut cloth, and even trimmed beards with iron shears like these.

Thick fleece shed once a year, in spring

Two sickle blades

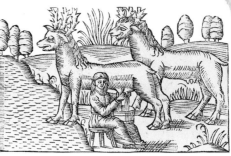

MILKING REINDEER
This 16th-century Swedish engraving shows a woman milking reindeer. In the far north, people farmed reindeer for their milk, meat, and hides. They were also hunted in many places, including Greenland (pp. 20–21).

BLACK SHEEP
Hebridean sheep were farmed by Vikings on the Hebrides islands. Like Manx Loghtan sheep (p. 37), they shed their wool naturally, and do not have to be sheared. They can live on sparse vegetation and are very hardy.

Ard blade

HARVEST TOOLS
The ground was broken up in the spring with an ard, a simple plough. Later grain was cut with iron sickles with wooden handles. The blades of these tools were sharpened with whetstones.

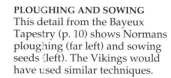

PLOUGHING AND SOWING
This detail from the Bayeux Tapestry (p. 10) shows Normans ploughing (far left) and sowing seeds (left). The Vikings would have used similar techniques.

FLOUR POWER
Grain was ground into flour with a quern stone. This one comes from a Viking farm at Ribblehead in Yorkshire, England. The grain was placed on the bottom stone. Then the top stone was laid on it and the wooden handle was turned around. Rich Vikings preferred finer flour, ground with querns made of lava imported from the Rhineland in Germany.

Top stone

Bottom stone

Ears and grains of spelt wheat

GRAINS
Spelt is an early form of wheat. The Vikings also grew barley and rye.

Ground wheat

LONGHORN COW
Cattle like this were once farmed in many parts of the Viking world. Now new breeds have been developed, and longhorn cattle only survive on a few special farms. Domestic animals weren't just raised for their meat and milk. Sheep's wool, cattle hide, and poultry feathers were also used to make clothes and bedding. Cattle horns are hollow, and are ideal as drinking horns. These were tricky to put down, and had to be rested in special holders. Animal bones were carved into knife handles, combs, pins, needles, even jewellery.

Getting around

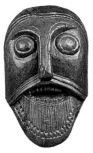

MUCH OF SCANDINAVIA is rugged and mountainous. The large forests, lakes, and marshes make travelling difficult, especially in bad weather. Vikings went everywhere they could by ship. Travelling overland was often easiest in winter, when snow covered uneven ground and the many rivers and lakes froze over. People got about on sledges, skis, and skates. In deep snow, they wore snowshoes. Large sledges were pulled by horses. To stop the horses from slipping on the ice, smiths nailed iron crampons (studs) to their hooves. In the summer, Vikings rode, walked, or travelled in wagons pulled by horses or oxen. Roads stuck to high land, to avoid difficult river crossings. The first bridge in Scandinavia, a huge wooden trestle, was built near Jelling in Denmark around the year 979, probably on orders from King Harald Bluetooth.

WELL GROOMED
A complete wooden wagon was found in the Oseberg burial ship (pp. 54–57). It is the only one known from Viking times. The surface is covered in carvings, including four heads of Viking men. The men all have well-groomed beards and moustaches.

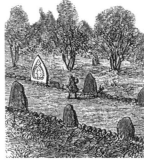

A GOOD DEED
Christian Vikings thought building roads and bridges would help their souls go to heaven. This causeway in Täby, Sweden was built by Jarlebanke (p. 59). He celebrated his good deed with a rune stone.

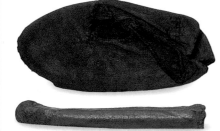

Bone ice skate from York, England

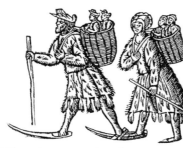

16th-century engraving of a Swedish couple skiing with single skis, as the Vikings did

ICE-LEGS
The word "ski" is Norwegian. Prehistoric rock carvings in Norway show that people have been skiing there for at least 5,000 years. The Vikings definitely used skis, though none have survived. Ice skates have been found all over the north. The Vikings called them "ice-legs". They were made by tying the leg bones of horses to the bottoms of leather boots. The skater pushed him or herself along with a pointed iron stick like a ski pole.

HORSING AROUND
Vikings were fine riders. This silver figure of a horseman comes from Birka in Sweden. It dates from the 10th century. The rider is wearing a sword, and must be a warrior.

Beech body decorated in iron studs with tinned heads

One of four carved animal heads

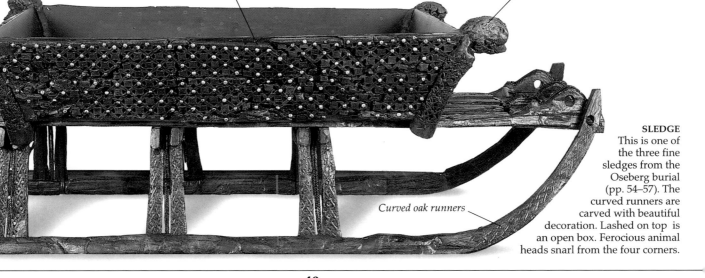

Curved oak runners

SLEDGE
This is one of the three fine sledges from the Oseberg burial (pp. 54–57). The curved runners are carved with beautiful decoration. Lashed on top is an open box. Ferocious animal heads snarl from the four corners.

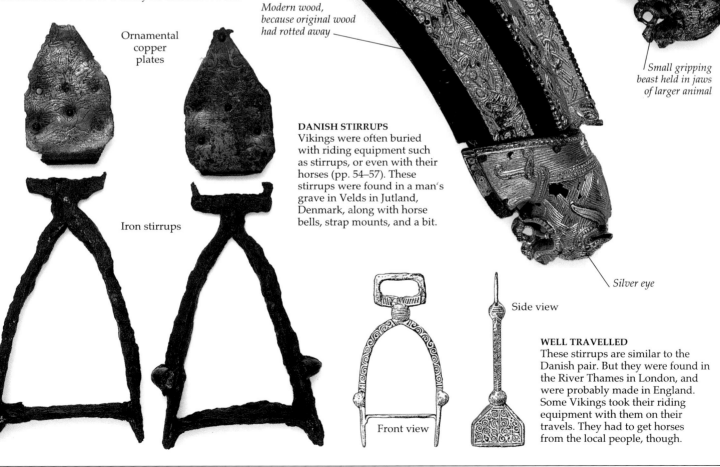

Copper alloy covered in gold

Hole through which reins passed

Ribbon decoration in Jellinge style

Animal heads, possibly meant to scare off evil spirits and stop horses from bolting

REINING THEM IN
Harness bows were only used in Denmark. The curved surface rested on a horse's back. The reins passed through the holes in the centre to stop them getting tangled up. This pair was found in a smith's hoard in Mammen, Jutland. They belonged to a wealthy chieftain, and were probably only used on ceremonial occasions. Their splendid decoration shows how wealthy he must have been.

Modern wood, because original wood had rotted away

Small gripping beast held in jaws of larger animal

Ornamental copper plates

Iron stirrups

DANISH STIRRUPS
Vikings were often buried with riding equipment such as stirrups, or even with their horses (pp. 54–57). These stirrups were found in a man's grave in Velds in Jutland, Denmark, along with horse bells, strap mounts, and a bit.

Silver eye

Side view

Front view

WELL TRAVELLED
These stirrups are similar to the Danish pair. But they were found in the River Thames in London, and were probably made in England. Some Vikings took their riding equipment with them on their travels. They had to get horses from the local people, though.

In the workshop

THE VIKINGS PARTLY OWE THEIR SUCCESS to skilled craftsmen who made their strong weapons and fast ships. The weapon-smith who forged sharp swords, spears, and axes (pp. 14–15) was the most respected. But smiths also made all the iron tools for working metal and wood. They knew how to work different metals and how to decorate them with elaborate techniques. Smiths also produced everyday objects like locks and keys, cauldrons for cooking, and iron rivets for ships. Viking carpenters were also highly skilled. They made a wide range of objects, including ships. They knew exactly what wood to use for what purpose, and how to cut timber to give maximum strength and flexibility. They carved decoration on many objects, and sometimes painted them with bright colours. Most of the colours have faded now, but enough survive to give an idea of the original effect.

Moulding iron for making grooves or patterns on planks

PRESSED GOLD
This gold brooch from Hornelund in Denmark was made from a lead die. The jeweller pressed the die into a sheet of gold to create a pattern. Then he decorated the surface with gold wire and blobs or granules of gold. Only the richest chieftains or kings could afford such a beautiful brooch.

Twisted gold wire forms heart-shaped patterns

One of three heart-shaped loops made of strands of twisted gold wire

Granules of gold

Plant decoration shows influences from Western Europe, but the technique is purely Scandinavian

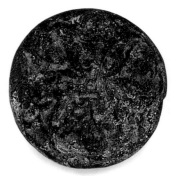

Lead die from Viborg, Denmark, used for making precious metal brooches like the Hornelund brooch

Plate shears for cutting sheet metal

Smith's tongs for holding hot iron on anvil

MAKING DRAGONS
Bronze was heated in a crucible over a fire until it melted. Then the smith poured it into the stone mould. When the metal cooled, he lifted out a fine dragon head with a curly mane. It may have decorated a fancy box. A stone mould like this one could be used over and over again. Many brooches and dress pins (pp. 48–49) were cast in similar moulds.

Modern casting

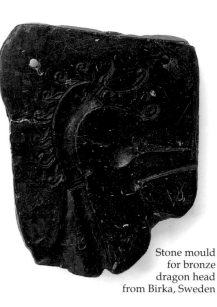

Stone mould for bronze dragon head from Birka, Sweden

Light hammerhead

Heavy hammer-head

HAMMERS
Hammers came in various weights. The heaviest were used for welding and forging swords, the lightest for delicate work like shaping wire.

Small detachable bit

Larger detachable bit, for boring bigger holes

AXES AND ADZES
The carpenter used an axe to fell (cut down) trees and chop off their branches. He then used a T-shaped axe (p. 15) to shape and smooth the planks. An adze has its blade at right angles to the handle. The carpenter could shape a log by chipping away at its surface with an adze.

Hole for wooden haft (handle)

Felling a tree with an axe

SHIP BUILDING
The Bayeux Tapestry (p. 10) shows how the Normans made ships. In the detail on the left, a man fells a tree. Above, a man trims a tree while another shapes the split trunks into planks with a T-shaped axe. Below, the planks are overlapped and riveted together. A carpenter smooths the planks. Another drills holes with a drill or auger, leaning against the curved end for extra force.

Adze head

SMITHING A SWORD
This carving is part of a 12th-century doorway from the church in Hylestad, Norway. It shows the hero Sigurd breaking a sword the smith Regin has made for him. In another scene (p. 51), Regin holds the hot iron with a pair of tongs and hits it against the anvil with a hammer. A helper works the bellows to keep the fire in the forge burning.

Wood is modern, as original wood had rotted away

The carpenter turned this T-shaped handle to bore the hole

A smith's tools
The tools on these two pages are part of a large hoard found in a chest at Mästermyr on the island of Gotland, Sweden. Their owner was a smith. He was able to work with sheet metal to make cauldrons and locks, but he could also cast, weld, and decorate bronze. He was a ship-builder, joiner, and wheelwright, and probably made the wooden tool chest as well!

A BORING TOOL
This drill or auger was used to make holes in planks, including rivet holes that held ship planks together. It had five bits of different sizes.

Back gives extra strength

BONE CUTTER
A small hacksaw could cut through bone and metal. The carpenter could also use its narrow blade for fine work.

Tang, a spike that used to fit into a wooden handle

WOOD SAW
The small lengths of wood needed to make buckets, boxes, and furniture were cut with this large saw.

Iron toothed blade

Shaped end for carpenter to lean on

Wooden handle

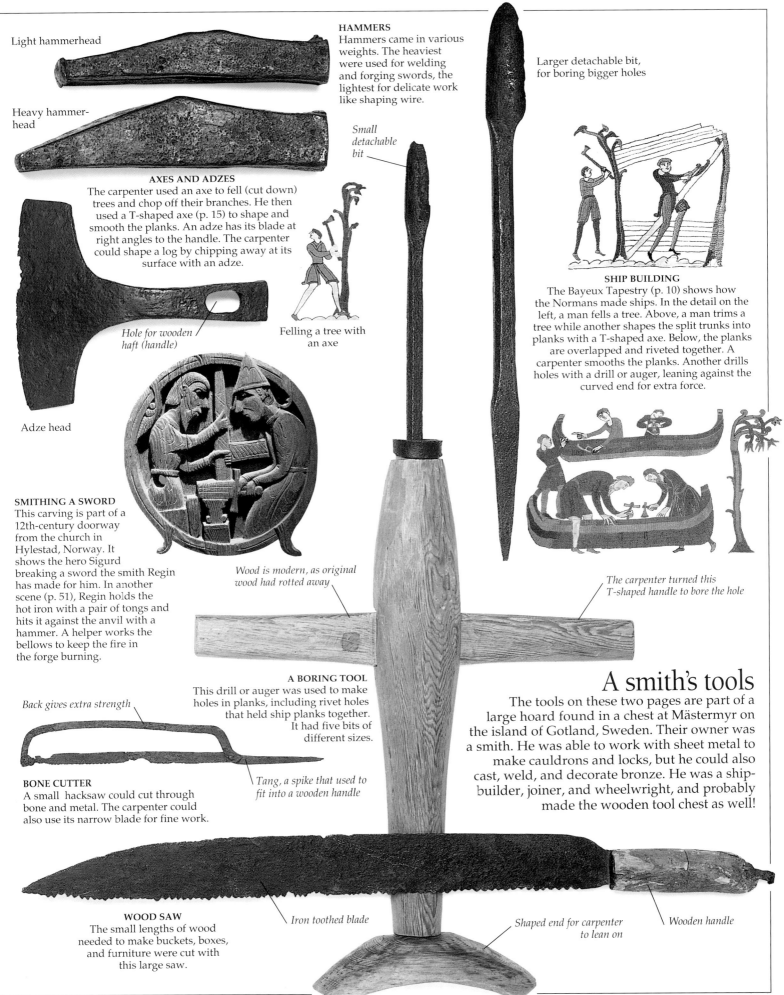

Spinning and weaving

ALL VIKING WOMEN (and probably some men) spent part of the day spinning wool or flax. Then they wove the family's clothes on a vertical loom which stood against the wall. Everyday clothes were cut from plain wool. But the borders of men's tunics and women's dresses were woven with geometric patterns, in bright colours or, for the very rich, gold and silver threads. Silk imported from far-off lands was made into hats and fancy borders for jackets. Fur trimmings on cloaks added a touch of style. Imitation fur was also fashionable.

Linen head cloth

Spindle whorl

SPINNING TOOLS
A spindle is a wooden rod used for spinning. It is passed through a spindle whorl, a round piece of clay or bone that makes the spindle spin with its weight. The weaver used rods called pin-beaters to straighten threads and make fine adjustments to the woven cloth.

Pin-beaters   Spindle

Wool being stretched and spun

Raw wool

Medieval woman spinning with raw wool held on a distaff

SPINNING A GOOD YARN
The spinner picks a tuft of raw wool from the basket and pulls it into a strand. She winds this around the spindle as it spins. When one tuft is spun, she adds the next tuft of wool to the strand.

Spun wool

Spindle whorl

Spindle

Brown silk

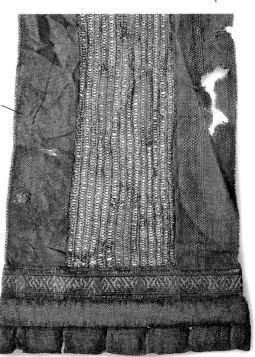

Raw, combed wool

FANCY CLOTHES
Fragments of a chieftain's clothes were found in a grave at Mammen, Denmark. They date from the late 10th century. This is the end of a long braid which the man may have used to fasten his cloak. It is made of silk, with gold embroidery on the borders. Animal figures and human faces also decorate the man's cloak and shirt. A reconstruction of his entire outfit can be seen on page 29. The beautiful Mammen Axe (pp. 6–7) was found in the same grave.

Cane basket

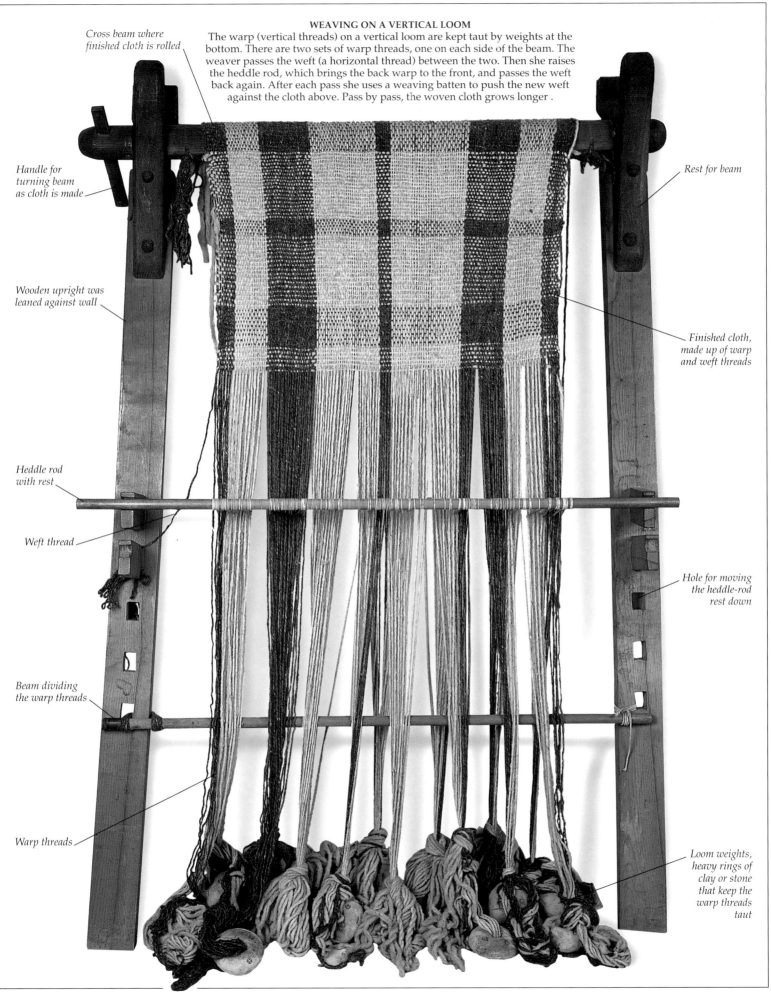

WEAVING ON A VERTICAL LOOM

The warp (vertical threads) on a vertical loom are kept taut by weights at the bottom. There are two sets of warp threads, one on each side of the beam. The weaver passes the weft (a horizontal thread) between the two. Then she raises the heddle rod, which brings the back warp to the front, and passes the weft back again. After each pass she uses a weaving batten to push the new weft against the cloth above. Pass by pass, the woven cloth grows longer .

Cross beam where finished cloth is rolled

Handle for turning beam as cloth is made

Wooden upright was leaned against wall

Heddle rod with rest

Weft thread

Beam dividing the warp threads

Warp threads

Rest for beam

Finished cloth, made up of warp and weft threads

Hole for moving the heddle-rod rest down

Loom weights, heavy rings of clay or stone that keep the warp threads taut

Jewellery

GOLD PENDANT
Women wore pendants on the end of necklaces. This thin piece of embossed gold was worn as a pendant. It was found in a hoard (p. 49) in Halton Moor, England.

THE VIKINGS LOVED BRIGHT ornaments. Their metalworkers were highly skilled at the intricate decoration of jewellery. Both men and women wore brooches, necklaces, finger-rings, and arm-rings (like bracelets). Wearing gold and silver jewellery was a sign of wealth and prestige. After a successful raid, a king might reward a brave warrior by giving him a prize piece. Bronze didn't shine as brilliantly as gold, but it was less expensive. Pewter, a mixture of silver and other metals, was cheaper still. The poorest Vikings carved their own simple pins and fasteners from animal bones left over after cooking. Coloured glass, jet, and amber were all made into pendants, beads, and finger-rings. Vikings also picked up fashions in jewellery from other countries and changed them to their own style.

Fine silver wires linked together as if they were knitted

SILVER ARM-RING
This massive arm-ring was found in Fyn in Denmark. It is solid silver, and must have weighed heavily on the arm. The surface is cut by deep, wavy grooves and punched with tiny rings and dotted lines. Four rows of beads decorate the centre. They look as if they were added separately, but the whole piece was made in a mould (p. 42).

RECYCLING
Vikings who settled abroad took their fashions with them. This gold arm-ring was made in Ireland. Vikings raided many Irish monasteries in search of precious metals. Sacred books and objects often had mounts made of gold and silver, which they ripped out and carried away. Later, smiths would melt the metals down and turn them into jewellery.

Animal heads

Gold wires of different thicknesses coiled together

SILVER SPIRAL
Spiral arm-rings could be worn high on the upper arm. They were only popular in Denmark, and were imported from the Volga area of Russia. This fine silver ring was found near Vejle in Jutland, Denmark.

IN ALL HIS FINERY
This tough Viking is wearing every imaginable kind of jewellery. His bulging biceps are being squeezed by spiral arm-rings in the form of snakes. But in many details, the old drawing is pure fantasy (p. 6).

THOR'S HAMMER...
Thor's hammer (pp. 7, 53) was often worn as a pendant, just like the Christian cross. Here animal heads at the ends of the chain bite the ring from which the hammer hangs.

Grooves are filled with niello, a black compound, to make them stand out

...AND A CROSS
An open, leafy pattern decorates this silver Christian cross. The cross and chain were found in Bonderup, Denmark. They were probably made around the year 1050.

Four double-twisted gold rods braided together

Danish necklace made of glass beads

NECKLACES AND RINGS

The Arab traveller Ibn Fadhlan (pp. 19, 55) met Viking women in Russia around 920. He wrote that "round the neck they have ornaments of gold or silver". These would have included neck-rings, which are stiff and inflexible, and necklaces, which can twist and bend. This gold neck-ring is the largest and most splendid ever found. It is solid gold and weighs over 1.8 kg (4 lb). It could only have been worn by a broad-chested man, because it is more than 30 cm (1 ft) wide! Many Viking neck-rings were made by melting down silver Arab coins. Glass made the brightest beads. Bead-makers started with imported glass or broken drinking glasses. They heated these up and fused them together to make beads with bright patterns and swirling mixtures of colours.

Silver neck-ring from Halton Moor, England, made of braided silver wires

A farmer in Tissø in Denmark found this massive gold neck-ring while ploughing a field

ARM-RING WITH TREES
This gold arm-ring from Råbylille in Denmark is stamped with some very fine decoration.

Tree

Cross

Gold ring from Denmark inscribed with runes (pp. 58–59)

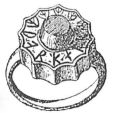

THREE GOLD RINGS
Finger-rings were made like miniature arm-rings. Both men and women wore them. But Swedish women were the only ones to wear ear-rings, which they dangled from chains looped over the ear.

Two gold finger-rings from Viking-age Ireland

Continued on next page

Brooches

Clasps and brooches were often lavishly decorated. But they weren't just for show. All Vikings wore brooches to hold their clothes in place. Women usually had two oval brooches to fasten their over-dresses (pp. 30–31). Men held their cloaks together with a single brooch on the right shoulder (pp. 28–29). In this way the right arm – the sword arm – was always free. Certain styles such as oval and trefoil brooches were popular all over the Viking world. Others, like the box brooches from Gotland, were only fashionable in certain areas.

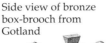

Heads covered in gold

Hair

Beard

Long moustache

Ears

Tin-coated ring and pin

One of four squatting human figures made of gold

Side view of bronze box-brooch from Gotland

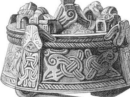

BOX BROOCH
Box brooches were shaped like drums. The magnificent brooch on the left comes from Mårtens on the island of Gotland, Sweden. A very wealthy woman wore it to fasten her cloak. The base is made of cast bronze, but the surface glitters with gold and silver.

MEN'S HEADS
The tips of this brooch from Høm in Denmark are decorated with three men's heads. Each face has staring eyes, a neat beard, and a long moustache. Brooches like this were first made in the British Isles. The Vikings liked them so much they made their own.

Top view of Mårtens box-brooch

Head of gripping beast

Head of slender animal

SHAPED LIKE CLOVER LEAVES
Trefoil brooches have three lobes. In the 9th and 10th centuries, women wore them to fasten their shawls. The finest ones were made of highly decorated gold and silver. Poorer women had simpler brooches, mass-produced in bronze or pewter. The trefoil style was borrowed from the Carolingian Empire to the south of Scandinavia, in what is now France and Germany.

Front view

Back view

GRIPPING BEASTS
Four gripping beasts (p. 37) writhe across this silver brooch made in Hunderup in Denmark. It was found at the site of Nonnebakken, one of the great Viking forts (pp. 22–23).

URNES AGAIN
The Urnes art style featured a snaky animal twisting and turning in dynamic coils (p. 36) It was the most popular decoration for 11th-century brooches, like this bronze one from Roskilde, Denmark.

THE PITNEY BROOCH
The Urnes art style was very popular in England and Ireland during the reign of Cnut the Great (1016–35). This beautiful gold brooch in the Urnes style was found at Pitney in Somerset, England.

Long pin would have been stuck through cloak

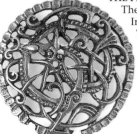

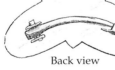

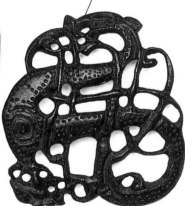

Bronze pin, possibly from a brooch, in Irish style but found in Norway

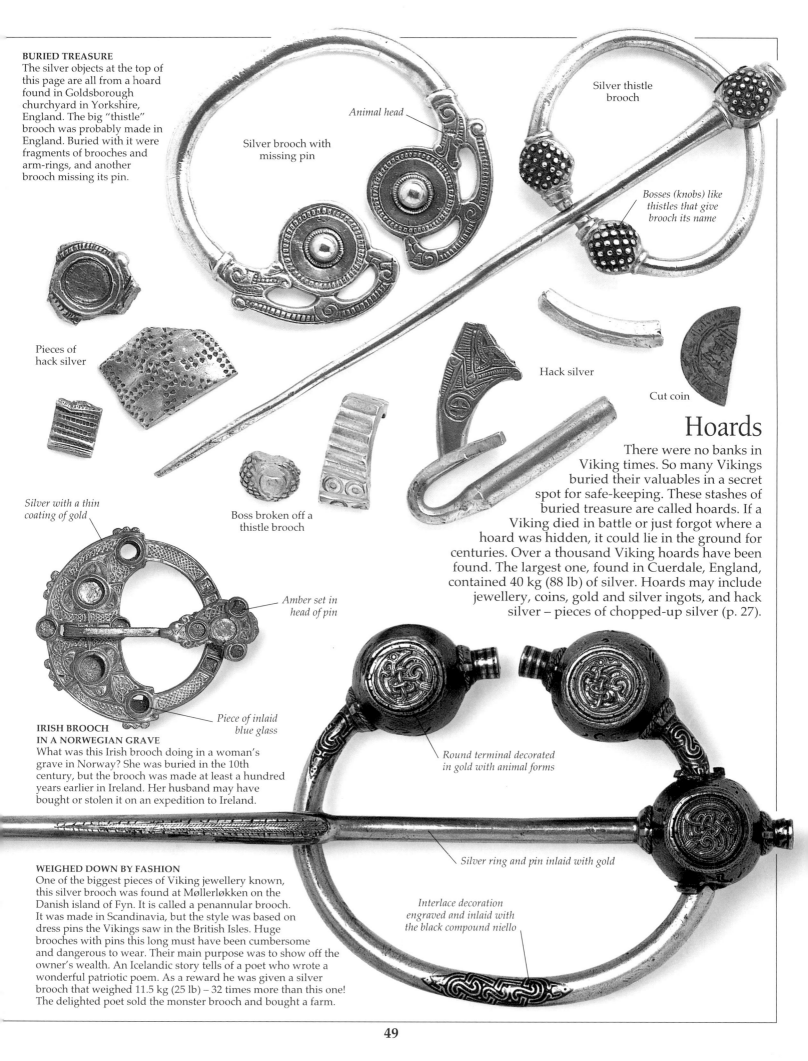

BURIED TREASURE
The silver objects at the top of this page are all from a hoard found in Goldsborough churchyard in Yorkshire, England. The big "thistle" brooch was probably made in England. Buried with it were fragments of brooches and arm-rings, and another brooch missing its pin.

Silver brooch with missing pin

Animal head

Silver thistle brooch

Bosses (knobs) like thistles that give brooch its name

Pieces of hack silver

Hack silver

Cut coin

Boss broken off a thistle brooch

Silver with a thin coating of gold

Amber set in head of pin

Hoards

There were no banks in Viking times. So many Vikings buried their valuables in a secret spot for safe-keeping. These stashes of buried treasure are called hoards. If a Viking died in battle or just forgot where a hoard was hidden, it could lie in the ground for centuries. Over a thousand Viking hoards have been found. The largest one, found in Cuerdale, England, contained 40 kg (88 lb) of silver. Hoards may include jewellery, coins, gold and silver ingots, and hack silver – pieces of chopped-up silver (p. 27).

Piece of inlaid blue glass

IRISH BROOCH IN A NORWEGIAN GRAVE
What was this Irish brooch doing in a woman's grave in Norway? She was buried in the 10th century, but the brooch was made at least a hundred years earlier in Ireland. Her husband may have bought or stolen it on an expedition to Ireland.

Round terminal decorated in gold with animal forms

Silver ring and pin inlaid with gold

Interlace decoration engraved and inlaid with the black compound niello

WEIGHED DOWN BY FASHION
One of the biggest pieces of Viking jewellery known, this silver brooch was found at Møllerløkken on the Danish island of Fyn. It is called a penannular brooch. It was made in Scandinavia, but the style was based on dress pins the Vikings saw in the British Isles. Huge brooches with pins this long must have been cumbersome and dangerous to wear. Their main purpose was to show off the owner's wealth. An Icelandic story tells of a poet who wrote a wonderful patriotic poem. As a reward he was given a silver brooch that weighed 11.5 kg (25 lb) – 32 times more than this one! The delighted poet sold the monster brooch and bought a farm.

Games, music, and stories

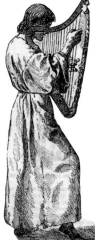

A FEAST WAS A TIME to relax. After they had eaten their full, Vikings played games, told stories, and listened to music. Kings had their own poets, called scalds, who entertained guests and praised the king. Stories and poems were told from memory and passed down from father to son. People knew all the exciting episodes by heart. Popular legends like Thor's fishing trip were carved on stone or wood (p. 58–59). Jesters and jugglers often amused the guests with tricks and funny dances. Some games were played on elaborate boards with beautifully carved pieces. Others were scratched on wood or stone. Broken pieces of pottery or scraps of bone could be used as counters. Many outdoor pastimes were the same as today. During the long winters, Vikings went skiing, sledging, and skating (p. 40). In the summer, they fished, swam, and went boating in the cold rivers and fjords.

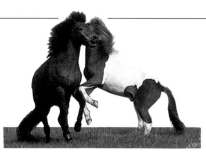

HORSE FIGHTING
These Icelandic ponies are fighting in the wild. Vikings enjoyed setting up fights between prize stallions (male horses). It was a serious matter, with bets laid on the winner. Horse-fighting may have played a part in religious feasts and ceremonies. The Vikings may have thought the winning horse was a special favourite of the gods.

SWEET HARP
In rich households, musicians played the harp or lyre to accompany stories and poems. Vikings were also keen singers. Talented singers would perform at feasts, and the whole assembly might join in a ballad or a popular folk song.

Such a horned headdress may have started the myth about Vikings wearing horned helmets

Blow here

BONE FLUTE
A Swedish Viking made this flute by cutting holes in a sheep's leg bone. He or she played it like a recorder, by blowing through one end. Covering the finger holes produced different notes.

Sound is produced as air passes this hole

Stave

Sword

Fingers cover bottom holes

Carved human head

Carved border decoration in Borre art style

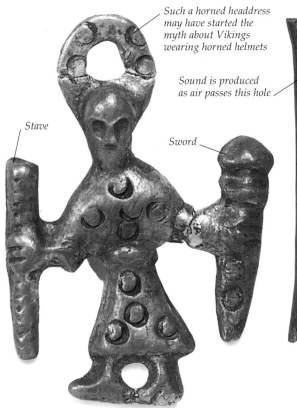

BALLINDERRY BOARD
A popular Viking board game was *hneftafl*. One player used his eight pieces to protect the king from the other player, who had 16 pieces. This wooden board from Ballinderry, Ireland may have been used for *hneftafl*. The central hole could have held the king.

Game pieces fit into 49 holes in board

DANCING GOD
This silver figure from Sweden may be a "dancing god". He is carrying a sword in one hand and a stave or spear in the other. Dancing was popular after feasts, and played a part in religious ceremonies. Some dances were slow and graceful. In the wilder ones, the dancers leapt about violently. After the coming of Christianity (pp. 62–63), priests tried to stop dancing altogether.

FIGURES OF FUN
Gaming pieces could be simple counters or little human figures. This amber man (far right) may have been the king in a game of *hneftafl*. He is holding his beard in both hands.

Two walrus ivory gaming pieces from Greenland

Amber gaming piece from Røholte, Denmark

Hands hold beard

In another part of the story, Sigurd's brother-in-law Gunnar tries to escape from a snake pit by playing a lyre with his toes and charming the snakes

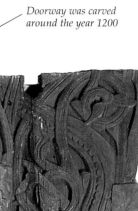

Doorway was carved around the year 1200

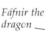

Fáfnir the dragon

Sigurd kills Fáfnir

Sigurd kills Regin

DOOM OF THE GODS

The Vikings told stories of *Ragnarök*, the "Doom of the Gods". This was a great battle between good and evil, when the gods would fight it out with horrible giants and monsters. The detail above comes from a 10th-century cross on the Isle of Man. It shows the god Odin (pp. 52–53) being eaten by the monstrous wolf Fenrir (p. 37).

Sigurd's horse Grani loaded with treasure

Sigurd tests the sword on the anvil and breaks it in two

Birds in a tree

The story starts with Regin forging Sigurd's sword

Sigurd sucks his thumb while cooking the dragon's heart

SIGURD THE DRAGON-SLAYER

The adventures of the hero Sigurd are carved on this wooden doorway from the church at Hylestad, Norway. Sigurd won fame and fortune by killing the dragon Fáfnir. The sword he used was forged by the smith Regin, who was the dragon's brother. But Regin was plotting to kill Sigurd and steal the treasure for himself. Some birds tried to warn Sigurd, but he couldn't understand them. Luckily he burned his hand cooking the dragon's heart and put his thumb into his mouth. One taste of the dragon's blood and Sigurd could understand the birds' twitterings. So he grabbed his sword and killed Regin.

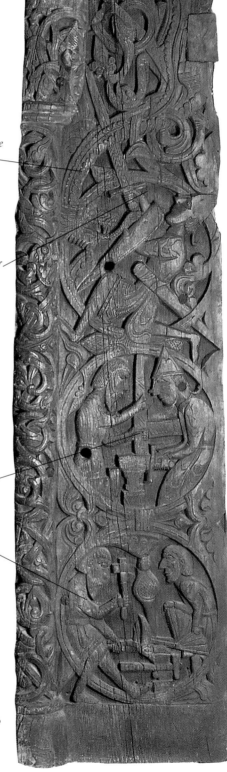

Gods and legends

Cone-shaped hat

THE VIKINGS BELIEVED IN MANY different gods and goddesses. The gods all had their own personalities, rather like human beings. The chief gods were Odin, Thor, and Frey. Odin, the god of wisdom and war, had many strange supernatural powers. Thor was more down-to-earth. He was incredibly strong, but he wasn't very clever. Frey, a god of fertility, was generous. The German traveller Adam of Bremen visited Uppsala in Sweden in 1075. He saw a great temple with statues of Odin, Thor, and Frey. Earlier in the Viking Age, people worshipped outdoors, in woods or mountains or by springs or waterfalls.

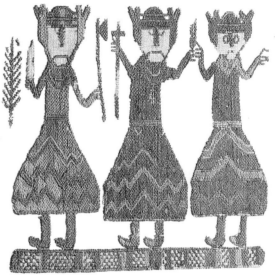

One hand holding beard, a symbol of growth

THREE GODS?
These three figures have been identified as Odin (left), Thor (middle), and Frey (right). But they may be kings or Christian saints. They are on a 12th-century tapestry from Skog church in Sweden (p. 63).

GODLY FAMILY
Frey was a god of fertility and birth. The best image of him is this small statue from Södermanland in Sweden. It is only 7 cm (3 in) high. People called on Frey in the spring for rich crops. When they got married, they asked Frey to bless them and give them many children. His sister Freyja was a goddess of fertility and love. One story says that half the warriors killed in battle went to join Freyja, while the rest went to Odin.

MONSTROUS MASK
Frightening faces were sometimes drawn on memorial stones or pieces of jewellery (p. 7). They may be gods, or they might have been meant to scare off evil spirits. This face from a stone in Århus, Denmark has a long braided beard and glaring eyes.

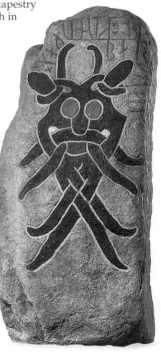

HIS LIPS ARE SEALED

Loki was part god and part devil. He could change his shape, and was always getting into mischief. In one story, Loki made a bet with a dwarf that he was a better metalworker. While the dwarf was heating up the furnace with bellows, Loki tried to distract him by turning into a fly and stinging him. But the dwarf won the bet anyway. To punish Loki and keep him quiet, he sewed his lips together. This stone bellows-shield shows Loki with his lips sewn up.

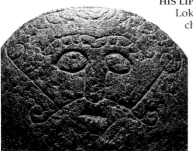

Silver Thor's hammer from Denmark

THOR'S HAMMER

Thor was popular with peasants and farmers. He rode through the sky in a chariot pulled by goats. There are many stories of his battles against evil giants and monsters, which he clubbed to death with his mighty hammer (p. 7).

A HERO'S WELCOME

The Valkyries were warrior women who searched battle-fields for dead heroes. They carried warriors who had died bravely to Valhalla, the Viking heaven. Here Odin welcomed the dead heroes, joining them in feasts in the great hall every evening.

A GIANT TAKES A BRIDE

In one story, the giant Thrym stole Thor's hammer. He said he would only give it back if he could marry Freyja. So Thor dressed up as Freyja and went to the ceremony. He nearly gave himself away by drinking too much! When Thrym brought out the hammer to bless the bride, Thor grabbed it and killed him and all the giant guests.

Dead warrior

Curved roof of Valhalla

Valkyrie (left) and man with axe (right)

Valkyrie with drinking horn greets dead hero

Runic inscription

Sail and rigging

PICTURES OF VALHALLA

A hero arrives in Valhalla on this picture stone from Gotland (p. 58). He is riding Odin's eight-legged horse, Sleipnir. A Valkyrie holds up a drinking horn to welcome him. Under the curved roof of Valhalla, another Valkyrie gives a drinking horn to a man with an axe and a dog.

Hero riding the eight-legged horse Sleipnir arrives in Valhalla

Ship full of armed warriors

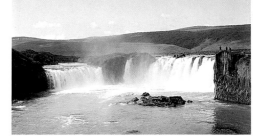

WATERFALL OF THE GODS

In Iceland, gods were worshipped at Godafoss, which means "waterfall of the gods".

TEARS OF GOLD

Freyja married a god called Od, who left her. All the tears she wept for him turned to gold. In this romantic picture, she is searching the sky for him in a chariot pulled by cats.

Viking burials

BEFORE THE COMING of Christianity, Vikings were buried with everything they would need in the next world. Traditional ceremonies varied a lot, and much is still shrouded in mystery. The wealthiest men and women were buried in ships, to carry them to the next world. These were crammed full of their belongings, from clothes and weapons to kitchen goods and furniture. Horses, dogs, even servants were killed and laid to rest with the dead Viking. The ships were then covered with mounds of earth, or set alight in a blazing funeral pyre. There are stories about burning ships being pushed out to sea, but there is no proof that this ever really happened. Other Vikings were placed in underground chambers in burial mounds. Even poor peasants were buried with their favourite sword or brooch.

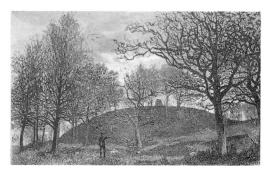

BURIAL MOUND
Amazing riches have been dug out of some burial mounds. Entire ships have survived in the right soil conditions. Even when the wood has disintegrated, the ship's outlines may be left in the earth. A ship from a mound in Ladby on Fyn, Denmark has been traced in this way. Many mounds contain burial chambers, not ships.

Prow ends in snake's head

Intricate carvings of lively animals

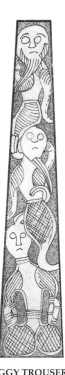

BAGGY TROUSERS
Three acrobatic human figures are carved inside the prow of the Oseberg ship. They have long, wispy beards and are doing strange gymnastics in baggy trousers.

Strakes get narrower towards the prow

Twelve strakes, each overlapping the one below

Stem is a single piece of fine oak, joined to keel at base

THE OSEBERG SHIP
The most beautiful Viking ship of all is the Oseberg ship. It was discovered in 1903 in a burial mound in Oseberg near the Oslo Fjord in Norway. Like the Gokstad ship (pp. 8–9), it had been preserved by the soggy blue clay of the fjord. This is the fine oak prow, or stempost. It is a modern copy, because only fragments of the original were left in the mound. Like the stern-post, it is carved with a brilliant array of animals and people. The prow ends in a curling snake's head, and the tip of the stern is the snake's tail. The ship is 21.5 m (70 ft 6 in) long and has 15 oarports (holes) on each side. As many as 30 men were needed to row it. But the Oseberg ship is a frail vessel that couldn't have sailed the open ocean. It was probably only used for state occasions or sailing up and down the coast. A mass of ship's equipment, including a gangplank, bailing bucket, mast, rudder, steering oar, anchor, and 15 pairs of oars, was found inside.

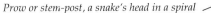

Prow or stem-post, a snake's head in a spiral

INSIDE THE BURIAL SHIP

The Oseberg ship is the most sumptuous Viking burial. The bones of two women were found inside. They had been buried in the mid 9th century. Judging by the rich furnishings, one was probably a queen. The other may have been her slave or servant. The ship also contained a richly carved wooden wagon, three beautiful sledges (p. 40), a work-sledge, and many pieces of furniture, tapestries, and kitchen utensils such as an iron cooking cauldron (p. 35). The carving on some of these objects is superb. The dead women must have once lain on the beds found in the burial chamber. These were littered with feathers, and other remains of bedding. Two oxen and at least 10 horses had also been slaughtered and thrown into the ship.

REBUILDING THE OSEBERG SHIP

The Oseberg burial mound was 44 m (144 ft) long and 6 m (20 ft) high. It was excavated in the summer of 1904. The ship inside was in very bad condition. It had been filled with heavy stones, which had broken the wood into thousands of fragments. Each one was numbered, washed, and protected with preservatives. Then the ship was painstakingly put back together, piece by piece.

Mast

Stern-post

Bailing bucket

Pine shield rack

Oars

Oarports (holes)

Hull of ship is made of oak

Keel, nearly 20 m (65 ft) long, made of two pieces of oak

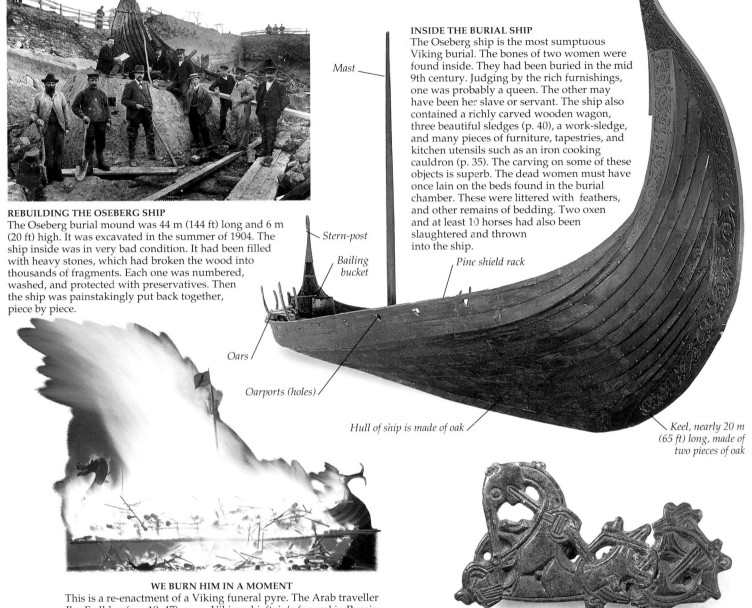

WE BURN HIM IN A MOMENT

This is a re-enactment of a Viking funeral pyre. The Arab traveller Ibn Fadhlan (pp. 19, 47) saw a Viking chieftain's funeral in Russia in 922. The dead man was dressed in beautiful clothes and seated in the ship, surrounded by drinks, food, and weapons. Then various animals and finally a woman were killed and laid in the ship with him. Then the ship was set on fire. Ibn Fadhlan was told: "We burn him in a moment and he goes at once to paradise".

BURIED BROOCH

No jewellery was found in the Oseberg ship, because the mound had been robbed long ago. But this bronze brooch was found in a woman's grave nearby. It is in the shape of an exotic animal with an arched head. The style is very similar to some of the Oseberg wood carvings.

BURIAL CHEST

The burial chamber of the Oseberg ship contained the fragments of many wooden chests. This is the best preserved one. It is made of oak wood decorated with broad iron bands. The elaborate locking system includes three iron rods that end in animal heads. The chest was full of tools, which the dead woman may have needed to repair her vehicles in the next world.

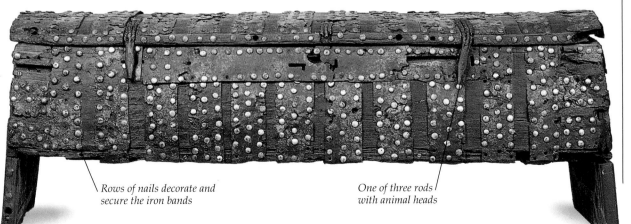

Rows of nails decorate and secure the iron bands

One of three rods with animal heads

Continued on next page

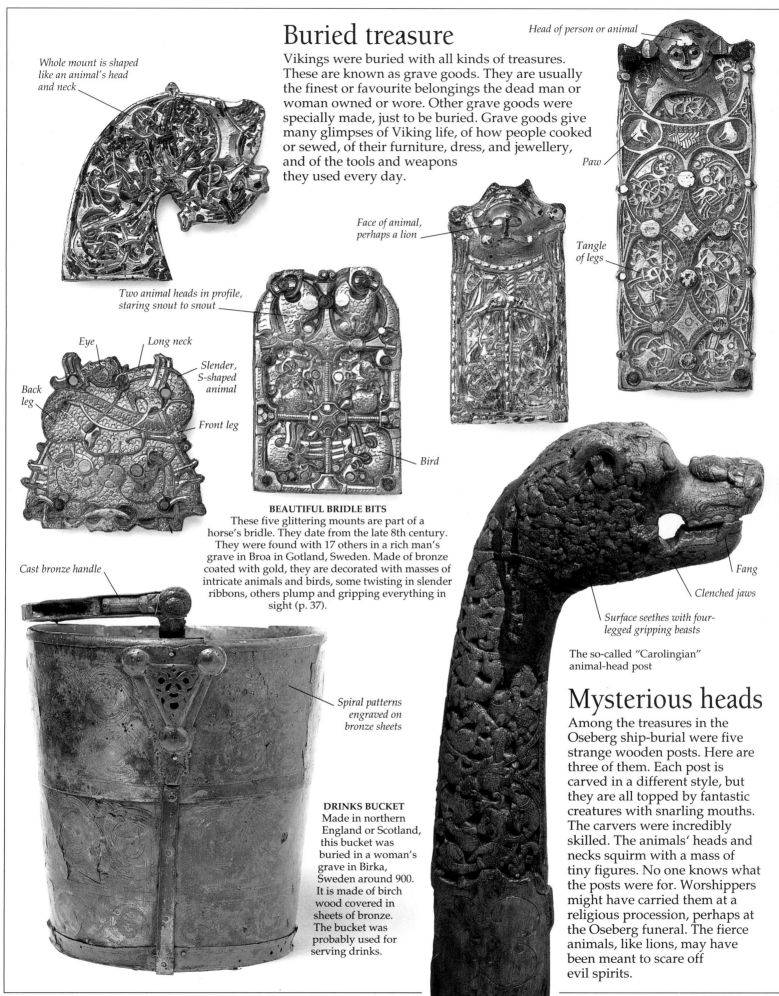

Buried treasure

Vikings were buried with all kinds of treasures. These are known as grave goods. They are usually the finest or favourite belongings the dead man or woman owned or wore. Other grave goods were specially made, just to be buried. Grave goods give many glimpses of Viking life, of how people cooked or sewed, of their furniture, dress, and jewellery, and of the tools and weapons they used every day.

Whole mount is shaped like an animal's head and neck

Head of person or animal

Paw

Tangle of legs

Face of animal, perhaps a lion

Two animal heads in profile, staring snout to snout

Eye

Long neck

Slender, S-shaped animal

Back leg

Front leg

Bird

BEAUTIFUL BRIDLE BITS
These five glittering mounts are part of a horse's bridle. They date from the late 8th century. They were found with 17 others in a rich man's grave in Broa in Gotland, Sweden. Made of bronze coated with gold, they are decorated with masses of intricate animals and birds, some twisting in slender ribbons, others plump and gripping everything in sight (p. 37).

Cast bronze handle

Spiral patterns engraved on bronze sheets

Fang

Clenched jaws

Surface seethes with four-legged gripping beasts

The so-called "Carolingian" animal-head post

Mysterious heads

Among the treasures in the Oseberg ship-burial were five strange wooden posts. Here are three of them. Each post is carved in a different style, but they are all topped by fantastic creatures with snarling mouths. The carvers were incredibly skilled. The animals' heads and necks squirm with a mass of tiny figures. No one knows what the posts were for. Worshippers might have carried them at a religious procession, perhaps at the Oseberg funeral. The fierce animals, like lions, may have been meant to scare off evil spirits.

DRINKS BUCKET
Made in northern England or Scotland, this bucket was buried in a woman's grave in Birka, Sweden around 900. It is made of birch wood covered in sheets of bronze. The bucket was probably used for serving drinks.

THE ENGLISH WAY

In their homes in Scandinavia, the Vikings raised huge memorial stones to remember dead friends or relatives (pp. 58–59). These stood in public places, often far from the dead person's grave. But in their colonies in England, the Vikings adopted the native custom of gravestones. This fragment of a stone from Newgate (near York) is decorated with two animals, one devouring the other. Traces of red paint show that it was once brightly coloured.

Head of first animal

SHIPS IN STONE

Only the very rich could afford a real ship to carry them to the next world. Other Vikings had their graves marked with raised stones in the shape of a ship. These ship settings are common all over Scandinavia. This is one of a whole fleet of ships in the big graveyard at Lindholm Høje in Jutland, Denmark.

PLANTS AND ANIMALS

These twisting figures decorate an 11th-century English gravestone. Two animals with S-shaped bodies form a figure-of-eight pattern. Plant leaves and shoots sprout from their snaky bodies.

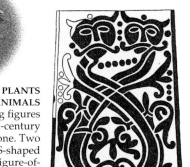

Second animal swallowing the first

Large glaring eyes

Swirling circles carved in very high relief

Flaring nostrils

Two elegant, intertwining animals

Metallic fangs and eyes

Surface decorated with hundreds of nails with heads shaped like flowers

Open jaw with large bared teeth

The "First Baroque" animal-head post

The "Academician's" animal-head post

All five posts had long wooden planks attached to their bases with wooden dowels

VIKING SOAP OPERA

This romantic painting shows the funeral pyre of Sigurd the dragon-killer (pp. 51, 58) and Brynhild (p. 30). In the legend, Sigurd was in love with Brynhild. But he married another woman instead and tried to trick Brynhild into marrying his brother-in-law, Gunnar. Brynhild was so angry that she had Sigurd killed. Overcome with grief, she stabbed herself and joined Sigurd on his funeral pyre.

Runes and picture stones

Vikings celebrated bravery in battle and the glory of dead relatives by raising memorial stones. These were carved with pictures and writing in runic letters (runes), often inside an intricate border of snakes. Some stones were raised by people who wanted to show off their own achievements. Others tell of loved ones who died on far-off voyages. The stones were set up in public places where many people could stop and admire them. The unusual picture stones from the island of Gotland often have no runes. But they are crowded with lively scenes of gods, ships, and warriors.

Sigurd's horse

Birds

Sigurd sucks his thumb

Dragon Fáfnir

Headless body of Regin

Sigurd kills dragon

SIGURD THE DRAGON KILLER
The complete legend of Sigurd (p. 51) is carved on a great rock at Ramsund in Sweden. The carver has cleverly fitted clues about all the episodes into the frame made of snakes. He has also turned one of the serpents into the dragon Fáfnir.

Warrior killed in battle

The eight-legged horse Sleipnir carries Odin through the sky

A JUMBLE OF PICTURES
This picture stone from Ardre, Gotland is a jumble of pictures. But several stories can be picked out. At the top, Odin's mysterious eight-legged horse, Sleipnir, carries the god across the sky. Below is a Viking ship, surrounded by episodes from the bloody story of Völund the blacksmith. He was taken prisoner by King Nidud. In revenge, Völund cut off the heads of both of the king's sons and made their skulls into cups. In the end, Völund escaped by forging a pair of wings and flying away. The small boat below the ship may be the god Thor fishing with the giant Hymir. According to the legend, Thor caught the World Serpent. But Hymir was so terrified that he cut the line.

Ship full of warriors, with large rectangular sail

May be Thor and Hymir fishing from small boat

The bird may be Völund flying away

Two figures fishing

Many other pictures cannot be identified with certainty

The large piece of limestone was carved and painted in the 8th century

Interlace border

Headless bodies of the king's two sons

Völund's forge with his hammer and tongs

Wild beast, perhaps a wolverine

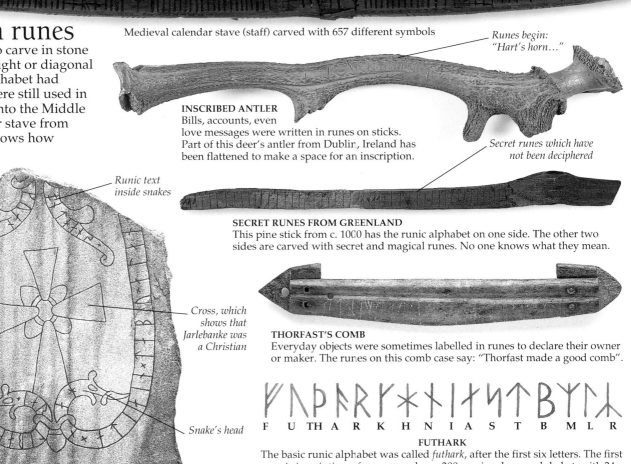

Medieval calendar stave (staff) carved with 657 different symbols

Writing in runes

Runes were easy to carve in stone or wood, with straight or diagonal lines. The basic alphabet had 16 runes. Runes were still used in Scandinavia well into the Middle Ages. The calendar stave from Sweden (above) shows how they developed.

Runes begin: "Hart's horn…"

INSCRIBED ANTLER
Bills, accounts, even love messages were written in runes on sticks. Part of this deer's antler from Dublin, Ireland has been flattened to make a space for an inscription.

Secret runes which have not been deciphered

SECRET RUNES FROM GREENLAND
This pine stick from c. 1000 has the runic alphabet on one side. The other two sides are carved with secret and magical runes. No one knows what they mean.

Snake's tail

Runic text inside snakes

Cross, which shows that Jarlebanke was a Christian

Snake's head

THORFAST'S COMB
Everyday objects were sometimes labelled in runes to declare their owner or maker. The runes on this comb case say: "Thorfast made a good comb".

F U TH A R K H N I A S T B M L R

FUTHARK
The basic runic alphabet was called *futhark*, after the first six letters. The first runic inscriptions, from around A.D. 200, are in a longer alphabet, with 24 characters. Around the year 800, the Viking alphabet with eight fewer runes was developed. Most inscriptions on stone were in normal runes. Another version of the alphabet was used for everyday messages on wood or bone.

SHOWING OFF
Jarlebanke was a wealthy 11th-century landowner who thought a lot of himself. He built a causeway over marshy land at Täby in Sweden. Then he raised four rune stones, two at each end, to remind travellers of his good deed. He also had this stone erected in the churchyard of Vallentuna, a village nearby. The runes say: "Jarlebanke had this stone raised in memory of himself in his lifetime, and made this Thing place, and alone owned the whole of this Hundred". The "Thing place" was the spot where the assembly for the district met (pp. 28–29). A Hundred was the area governed by a Thing.

SAINT PAUL'S STONE
In 1852, the end slab of a splendid tomb was found in the churchyard of St Paul's Cathedral in London, England. The whole tomb must have been shaped like a box. This is a colour painting of the great beast (p. 56) that decorates the slab. The colours are based on tiny traces of pigment found on the stone. The beast is very dynamic, twisting and turning around a smaller animal. The decoration shows that it was carved in the 11th century. The runes on the edge of the slab say: "Ginna and Toki had this stone set up". These two may have been warriors in Cnut the Great's army. Cnut became King of England in 1016 (p. 63).

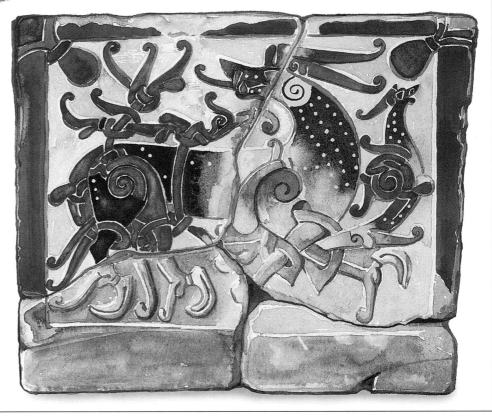

The Jelling Stone

THE GREATEST STONE MONUMENT in Scandinavia is the Jelling Stone. It was raised by King Harald Bluetooth at the royal burial place of Jelling in Jutland, Denmark. Beside the stone are two huge mounds. One of these, the North Mound, may be where Harald's parents, King Gorm and Queen Thyre, were buried in a traditional ceremony (pp. 56–57). When Harald became a Christian, he built a church next to the mounds and had his parents re-buried inside. Then he raised the Jelling Stone in their memory. The memorial also advertised his own power as king of Norway and Denmark. This a modern copy of the stone. It is a three-sided pyramid, with a long inscription on one side and pictures on the other two.

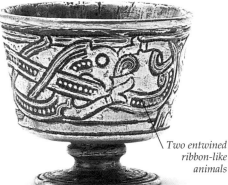

SILVER MOUNT
King Gorm may have worn this mount on his belt. It was found in a grave in the church in Jelling, among the re-buried bones of a man, probably Gorm.

Two entwined ribbon-like animals

GORM'S CUP?
This silver cup, usually known as the Jelling Cup, was found in the North Mound. It is no bigger than an eggcup. King Gorm may have drunk fruit wine from it. The cup is decorated with ribbon-like animals that gave their name to a style of Viking art, the Jellinge style.

Original stone is a single, massive boulder of red-veined granite

The great beast, a wild animal with sharp claws and a long tail

The beast is entwined in the coils of a huge snake

Ribbon-like decoration in the Mammen style, a development of the Jellinge style seen on the cup, with the ribbons based on plants rather than animals

Runes here continue from the inscription on the first side, reading: "…and Norway…"

GREAT BEAST
One side of the stone is carved with a snake twisting and turning around a great animal. Their struggle may represent the battle between good and evil. The animal could be a lion, but it is often just called "the great beast". It became a popular image in Viking art, and can be seen on weather vanes (p. 9) and rune stones like the St Paul's Stone (p. 59)

A ribbon forms a
border to the carving

These bright
colours are only a
guess, because the
original pigment
has disappeared

Halo, a symbol of
Christ's holiness

Christ with
outstretched
arms

Carvings are
in low relief

Plant leaves and shoots spring
from the ends of the ribbon

Horizontal lines of
runes cut into stone

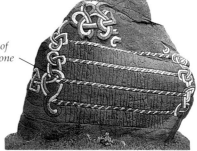

HARALD'S INSCRIPTION
One side of the Jelling Stone is
covered in runes. They read: "King
Harald commanded this memorial
to be made in memory of Gorm,
his father, and in memory of
Thyre, his mother – that Harald
who won the whole of Denmark
for himself, …". The inscription
continues beneath the great
beast and on below Christ.

More plant-like
ribbons wrap
around Christ

Harald's inscription
ends beneath the
figure of Christ with:
"…and made the
Danes Christian".

**BEARDED
CHRIST**
The third side
of the stone is
carved with the
oldest picture of Christ
in Scandinavia. Christ's
arms are outstretched, as if he
was on the cross, but no cross is
actually shown. Harald was converted to
Christianity around 960. He was influenced
by a miracle performed by the monk Poppo.
But he also converted for political reasons, to
strengthen his kingdom and to make sure that
Denmark could trade with Christian countries.

The coming of Christianity

SCANDINAVIA WAS SURROUNDED by Christian countries. Viking traders often wore crosses so they could travel freely through Christian lands (p. 27). But most Vikings remained loyal to the old gods until late in the 10th century. Then kings started supporting missionaries from England and Germany because they saw Christianity as a way to strengthen their power. Denmark was converted under King Harald Bluetooth in the 960s. Norway followed early in the 11th century. In Sweden, the traditional beliefs survived until the end of the 11th century (p. 52). The Vikings finally gave the old gods up when they saw that kings or missionaries who destroyed their statues were not punished by Odin, Thor, or Frey.

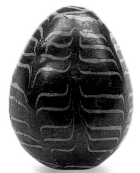

RESURRECTION EGG
This colourful egg was a symbol of Christ's resurrection. It was made in Russia, and may have been brought to Sweden by Russian missionaries.

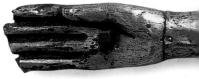

THE CHURCH AND THE SWORD
King Olaf Haraldsson turned Norway into a Christian country around 1024. He had old temples destroyed and forced people to convert.

STAVE CHURCH
Wooden churches were put up all over Scandinavia as soon as the people converted to Christianity. They were built like Viking houses, with wooden staves (planks) set upright in the ground. The first stave churches were simple, one-storey buildings. By the 12th and 13th centuries, elaborate churches with many roofs were being built. This is the stave church from Gol in Norway, built around 1200, and now in the Folk Museum in Oslo.

Spire

Turret

Gables decorated with carved dragon heads like ones on reliquary

More carved dragons

Portals are all crowned with crosses

Roofed-in verandah that runs right around church

LIKE A LITTLE CHURCH
Just like a miniature church, this little shrine or reliquary is decorated with dragon heads. Reliquaries were built to hold holy Christian relics. This one was made for Eriksberg church on Gotland, Sweden, in the late 1100s. Four little animal paws hold it up. The reliquary glitters with a thin layer of gold, over its frame of carved wood. It probably once held bones or fragments of cloth that people believed came from the body or clothes of a saint.

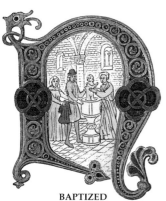

BAPTIZED
Baptism in water was a true sign of conversion. People wore the white baptismal clothes for a week after the ceremony.

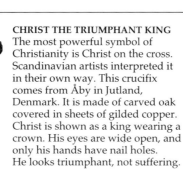

CHRIST THE TRIUMPHANT KING
The most powerful symbol of Christianity is Christ on the cross. Scandinavian artists interpreted it in their own way. This crucifix comes from Åby in Jutland, Denmark. It is made of carved oak covered in sheets of gilded copper. Christ is shown as a king wearing a crown. His eyes are wide open, and only his hands have nail holes. He looks triumphant, not suffering.

CNUT THE GREAT
Born in Denmark, Cnut invaded England in 1016. By 1028, he was king of Denmark, England, and Norway. Though he took England by the sword, he was a Christian king who built churches to make up for the bloody raids of his Viking ancestors.

Collar

Hair hangs down in long braids

Only hands are nailed to cross

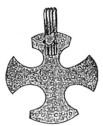

Early Scandinavian cross from Birka in Uppland, Sweden

Knee-length tunic tied in place with cords

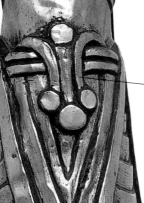

AWAY, DEVILS!
Ringing church bells to call people to church was an important sign of official Christianity. These bell-ringers are woven on a 12th-century tapestry from Skog church in Sweden (p. 52). They are thought to be ringing the bells to keep the old gods away.

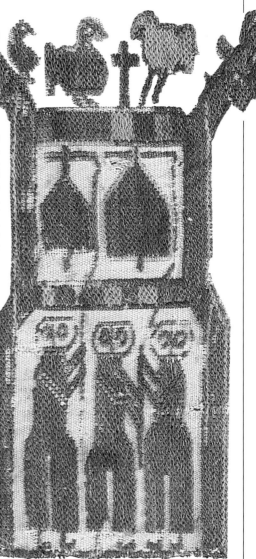

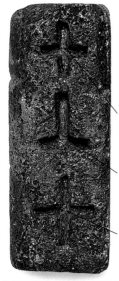

Cross

Thor's hammer

Cross

BEST OF BOTH WORLDS
The old gods did not die overnight. This stone mould from Himmerland in Denmark shows that craftsmen were happy to make Thor's hammers and Christian crosses at the same time. Many Christian Vikings kept their faith in Thor, just in case.

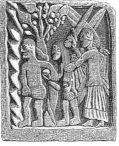

ADAM AND EVE
Scandinavian craftsmen soon started depicting scenes from the Bible as well as dragons and Viking legends. This stone carving from Skara church in Sweden shows Adam and Eve being expelled from Paradise.

Index

Acknowledgements

Dorling Kindersley would like to thank:
Birthe L. Clausen at the Viking Ship Museum, Roskilde, Denmark; Vibe Ødegaard and Niels-Knud Liebgott at the National Museum of Denmark, Copenhagen; Brynhilde Svenningsson at the Vitenskapsmuseet, Univ. of Trondheim, Norway; Arne Emil Christensen and Sjur H. Oahl at the Viking Ship Museum, Oslo, Norway; Lena Thalin-Bergman and Jan Peder Lamm at the Statens Historika Museum, Stockholm, Sweden; Patrick Wallace and Wesley Graham at the National Museum of Ireland, Dublin; Elizabeth Hartley at York Museum & Christine McDonnel & Beverly Shaw at York Archaeological Trust, England; Dougal McGhee; Claude & Mimi Carez; Niels & Elizabeth Bidstrup in Copenhagen and

Malinka Briones in Stockholm for their warm hospitality; Norse Film and Pageant Society; Helena Spiteri for editorial help; Manisha Patel and Sharon Spencer for design help.
Additional photography: Geoff Dann (models 12, 13, 19, 27, 28, 30, 31, 44 and animals 37, 38–39); Per E. Fredriksen (32bl, 32–33); Gabriel Hildebrandt at the Statens Historika Museum, Stockholm; Janet Murray at the British Museum, London.
Illustrations: Simone End, Andrew Nash
Index: Céline Carez

Picture credits
a=above, b=below, c=centre, l=left, r=right
Archeological & Heritage Picture Library, York: 16bc; Bibliothèque Nationale, Paris: 16br; Biofoto, Frederiksberg/Karsten Schnack: 20cl, /JK Winther: 22cr; Bridgeman Art Library, London/Jamestown-Yorktown Foundation/©M Holmes: 21tl, /Musée d'Art Moderne,

Paris/Giraudon, Wassily Kandinsky "Song of the Volga" 1906, © ADAGP, Paris and DACS, London 1994: 19br, /Russian Museum, St Petersburg, © Ilya Glazunov "The Grandsons of Gostomysl": 18bl; British Museum: 2bc, 4cal, 5bc, 6cr, 14c, 16cl, 25tr, 27cl, 29bl, 29br, 30bl, 36bc, 37cl, 46tl, 46c, 47c 2nd out, 47br, 48bl, 49tr, 59cr 4th down; Jean-Loup Charmet, Paris: 6tl, 10tl, 16c, 19tr, 34tl, 38br; DAS Photo: 55cl; CM Dixon: 12br, 52cr, /Museum of Applied Arts, Oslo: 13tl; Mary Evans Picture Library: 14cr, 17tc, 20tl, 30tl, 46cr, 53cl, 53br; Fine Art Photographs: 57bl, Forhistorisk Museum, Moesgård: 52br; Werner Forman Archive: 21tr, 24br, /Arhus Kunstmuseum, Denmark: 53tl, /Statens Historiska Museum: 52cr, 63br, /Universitetets Oldsaksamling, Oslo: 43cl; Michael Holford/Musée de Bayeux: 10bl, 15cr, 34tr, 34br, 35bl, 38bl, 38bc, 43tr, 43cr; Frank Lane Picture Agency/W Wisniewski: 50tr; Mansell Collection: 12bl, 50tl; Museum of London: 44tc, 44cr; © Nasjonalgalleriet, Oslo 1993/J Lathion: Christian Krohg "Leiv Eirikson discovering America" oil on canvas (313 x 470cm): 24tr, Johannes Flintoe

"The Harbour at Skiringssal" oil on canvas (54 x 65 cm) (detail): 28bl; National Maritime Museum: 24cal, /James Stephenson: 25car; Nationalmuseet, Copenhagen/Kit Weiss: 29tr, 29c, 44br; National Museum of Ireland: 7cr, 16tr, 17tr, 50cr, 59tr 2nd down; Peter Newark's Historical Pictures: 11cl, 17cl; Novosti /Academy of Sciences, St Petersburg: 22tr; © Pierpont Morgan Library, New York 1993 M736 f 9v: 7bl, f 12v: 17tl; Mick Sharp: 38tr; Statens Historiska Museum, Stockholm / Bengt Lundberg: 28tl; TRIP: 32tr, 57tl; Universitets Oldsaksamling, Oslo: 8tr, 9tl, 13tr, 13cl, 25tc, 32tr, 43cl, 51c, 55tl, 55tr, 55cr; Vikingeskibs-hallen Roskilde/Werner Karrasch: 11cl; Vitenkapsmuseet, University of Trondheim/ Per Fredriksen: 30cl, 32bl, 32/33b; Eva Wilson: 59br.

Every effort has been made to trace the copyright holders. Dorling Kindersley apologises for any unintentional omissions and would be pleased, in such cases, to add an acknowledgement in future editions.

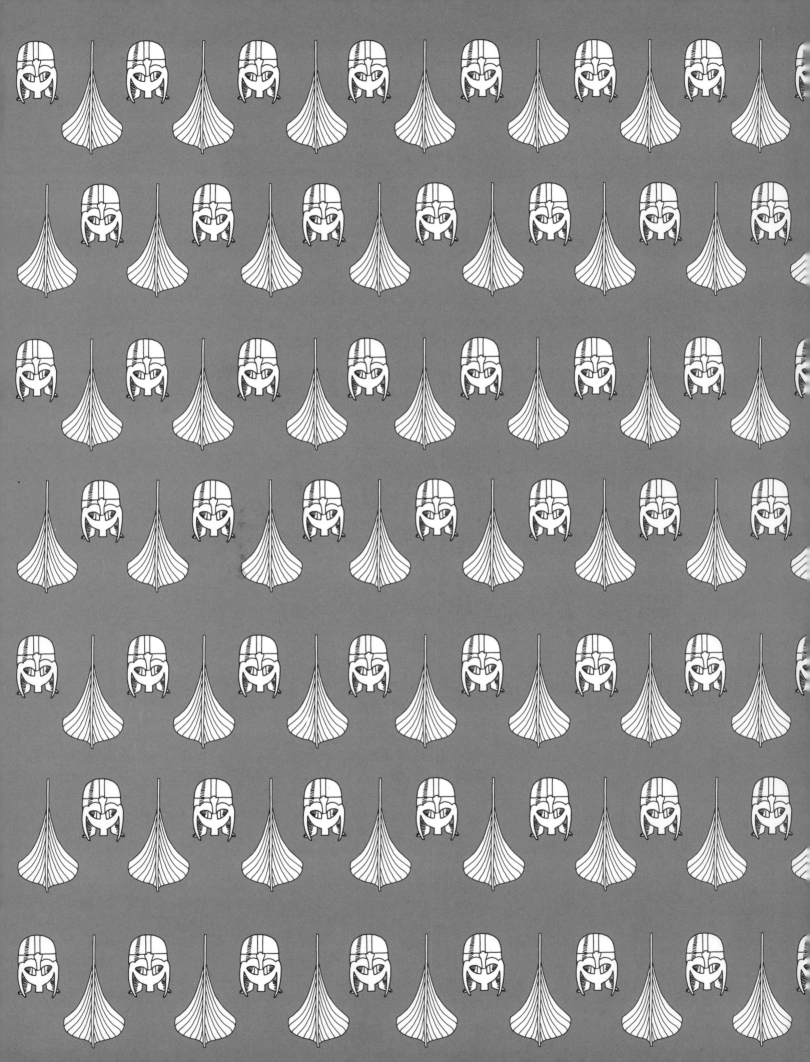